FOOTSTEPS TO SURVIVAL

FOOTSTEPS TO SURVIVAL

by
Michael F. Holodnak

Philosophical Library
New York

Library of Congress Cataloging in Publication Data

Holodnak, Michael F.
  Footsteps to survival.

    1. Holodnak, Michael F. 2. Hip joint—Surgery—Patients—United States—Biography. 3. Artificial hip joints—Complications and sequelae. 4. Hospitals, Veterans'—United States. I. Title.
RD549.H64 1984   617'.581059'0924 [B]   83-19393
ISBN 0-8022-2432-6

Copyright 1983 by Philosophical Library, Inc.
200 West 57th Street, New York, N.Y. 10019.
All rights reserved.

Manufactured in the United States of America.

Chapter 1

When I had my damaged hip joints replaced with artificial ones in a large Veterans Administration hospital, I did not perceive then that later I would be facing a continuous series of life-threatening disasters.

The complications were not so much from the botched-up hip surgery, as from my arthritis, the medication and the ponderous and indifferent hospital system which was geared to accommodate the staff members rather than the patients.

My ambulatory problem began a couple of years before the surgery. Prior to that, my arthritis was limited to only my rigid "bamboo spine," while the rest of my body joints were free of pain and inflammation. But when the inflammation reached my hip joints, despite all the anti-inflammatory drugs I was taking, the cartilages were gradually burnt away, leaving just bone rubbing against bone.

Getting up from a sitting position was tormenting and when I tried to walk I did so with a slow waddle, my painful hip joints crackling resoundingly. It was evident to me that my walking days were numbered.

For several months I had been going to a private arthritis specialist, Doctor H. Since my wife, Stephanie, was working in a factory during the day, I had been driving myself to Dr. H.'s office in New Haven whenever I had an appointment.

One day I parked my car in back of the building and painfully climbed the one flight of rickety stairs. Unassisted by a cane or crutches, I walked with a pronounced stoop to the waiting room.

When I finally got into Dr. H.'s office, he examined my hips and knees and asked me if I would mind going back to the V.A. hospital for intense physical therapy. I was already familiar with their less-than-an-hour-per-day therapy which I could just as easily do at home, so I declined his offer.

"Why?" he asked.

"Because I'm already doing the therapy at home with my wife's help. Also, I'm very busy writing a novel."

Dr. H.'s eyebrows went up and his eyes grew larger. "What's it about?"

"It's about modern industrial workers," I said.

"It sounds interesting," the doctor said. Then he got back to the subject at hand, and admitted that there was nothing more he could do for me to stop the inflammation.

Although in the back of my mind I was hoping he would come up with some magic cure, I had already seen the handwriting on the wall and was not too surprised to hear the stark truth that he could not help me.

I felt helpless and bitter, and said, " I guess I'm going to become a damn wheelchair case."

"No, you won't," he said.

Like a man reprieved from a death sentence, I stared at him. "What do you mean?" I said.

"We'll give you artificial hips," he said.

This was the first time I had heard of artificial hip joints and I left his office with my depressive pessimism immediately replaced with a dose of tentative hope.

A few days later, I received a phone call from Dr. H., who told me that a famous Ankylosing Spondylitis specialist would be in New Haven on May 7th, and asked me if I would be available for him to see me.

I immediately accepted the invitation and, after hanging up the phone, my mind went wild with anticipation and hope. A famous specialist might know more than Dr. H. did. Therefore, he might be able to do more for my poor hip joints, possibly even cure them altogether. I was vaguely aware of how foolish I was to believe that, but desperation often has a blinding effect on reason.

It was with this unreasonable attitude that Stephanie and I had driven to a major local hospital, talking like happy school kids about miracles, Stephanie smiling from ear to ear.

We got to the D. Building at 8 A.M., and a few minutes later, Dr. H. came to show us the way to the amphitheatre. There, in a small room next to the amphitheatre entrance, the famous specialist, an energetic, thin person with iron-gray hair, examined my knees and hips by manipulating my legs and talking in medical mumbo-jumbo to the few doctors that surrounded us, never saying a word to me, whom he probably regarded as a brainless specimen.

I managed to get the drift of his conversation with the doctors, which was that I was a well-motivated person who would be a good candidate for total hip replacement.

The specialist told me to wait there and went into the amphitheatre to lecture to a large audience of medical people sitting up in the round balcony.

I looked at Stephanie, who was no longer smiling. She asked me what they said. Even though she was sitting beside me she could not hear well because her hearing had become impaired from the high noise level at the plant where she worked.

I told her what I had heard, and she seemed disappointed. "He didn't tell you anything more than Dr. H. did," she said glumly.

We waited and listened through the small open door to sounds of the specialist who lectured and showed some slides with the lights dimmed.

When the lights went on again, I was called into the arena. The specialist asked me a few questions, in loud tones so his audience could hear him, and I answered also in loud tones.

Then he asked me to walk across the floor. As I did so, he verbally described the characteristics of an Ankylosing Spondylitis victim, whose peripheral joints had become affected; the stoop, the funny ambulation, the loud creaking sounds that could be heard by the people in the front rows.

The specialist thanked me, then dismissed me and went on with his lecture, and Stephanie and I left. It was a demeaning experience and I felt humiliated. On our journey toward home, Stephanie and I just stared ahead like a couple of clams.

Despite the medication I had been taking and the exercises I had been doing, my hip joints continued deteriorating. Each time I sat on or got up from a chair, my hip joints creaked like rusty hinges, and they were terribly painful.

However, once I was on my feet, I would soon become acclimated to the standing position and would be able to walk, amid a crescendo of clicking sounds, with only a moderate amount of pain. But because there was a lot of resistance in my leg motions, the walk would soon become very exhausting. Also, sleeping at night was difficult because the gnawing ache in my hips required frequent shifting of positions.

Although I still worked on my novel, I was otherwise totally disabled. I could not help Stephanie any more. She worked all day, then came home and made supper, washed dishes and clothes, and every evening helped me do my leg exercises. Though she was glad to do it, I could see that many evenings she was very tired, and the worse part of it was that I could do nothing but feel bad about it.

As much as I dreaded the surgery, I was now looking forward to it.

Dr. H. phoned to tell me that hip surgery was not done very often in this country. They had an English doctor teaching the technique to the doctors here who would then perform it on me. A special glue to hold the prosthesis in place had not yet been approved in this country by the Food and Drug Administration. He asked me to hold on for about four more months and to go back into the hospital to be evaluated and to have some more x-rays taken so that everything would be ready for the surgeons.

Reluctant as I was to return to the hospital, I decided that if I wanted to get better, I would have to do so, and I wondered what kind of whirlwind I was getting into.

In the admittance office, Stephanie and I were shuffled from one bureaucrat to another, and two and a half hours later, I was finally admitted.

In the ward, four doctors had examined the range of motion in my legs and said I was still in pretty good shape. They wanted me to keep exercising my legs so that the hip joints would not become fused, otherwise the surgery would be impossible to do.

I was later sent to the other building of the hospital, where an orthopedic surgeon examined my x-rays and my legs. Then he told me the discouraging news. He said that hip surgery was a very serious business and was not everything it was cracked up to be and could prove to be dangerous to the patient's very life. A lot of evaluation had to go into it before a person could become a candidate for it. It had been done in England for the past seven years, since 1965. But in this country, it could not be done on anyone under age fifty, except in extenuating circumstances, as in my case.

Every afternoon I went to Physical Therapy, where I soaked for about twenty minutes in a Hubberd whirlpool and then peddled the bicycle for a while. That was the extent of my "intensive therapy."

Again I had my hips, knees and chest x-rayed, then I went home on a two-day weekend pass.

After I returned to the hospital, another orthopedic surgeon came to examine me. He thought that "cups" would be better for me than the total hip replacement. He admitted that cups had their drawbacks and were good for only a few years. "But," he added brightly, "by then you would be old enough to get artificial hip joints."

Then I went with him to his office where we examined my x-rays. The irregular shape of the left femur head seemed less damaged than that of the right one, but I noticed a small hollow spot in the bone.

He told me it was a cyst that would have to be scraped away when they inserted the cups. He stressed the long recovery period and had a nurse escort me to see two patients who recently had cups put in.

The first patient had had both cups put in, one a few months earlier and the other, in the leg that was now in traction, three weeks ago. He told me it did not hurt him now, but in the first week it hurt him a lot.

The second patient I saw had one cup put in, but he had had a setback because calcium accumulated around it, causing him much pain when he moved that hip.

I was very unimpressed with the "cups," especially considering the long recovery period, with its confining pain and agony. I needed and I wanted help, but it was ridiculous for me to risk my life on either the artificial hips or the cups when both were of dubious value. It was a dilemma and I did not know what in hell to do!

In any event, when the surgeon asked me if I had made up my mind about the cups, I stupidly told him that since I did not have much choice, I would go with the cups.

Appearing pleased, the surgeon told me the surgery would take place either this week or the week after.

In the meantime, they sent me to radiology for even more hip x-rays, which were always a terrible experience for me.

I got to the x-ray room where a young female technician helped position me on the table. She wanted me to lie flat on my back with my legs straight. The table was hard and my spine protruded at the lumbar region and my hips were badly ankylosed, which made it impossible for me to do as she asked. She ignored my explanation and continued to insist that I had to do it. I asked her to get something soft to put under my spine. She said that she did not have time to look for anything.

Her black female assistant put her hand on my protruding spine, then placed a folded linen under it. Finally, I was able to lie flat and gradually got my legs straight. This same young lady then placed a pillow under my head to give me even more comfort. I was touched by her compassion and kindness, which was in sharp contrast to the other technician, who was only interested in getting her job done.

After taking one exposure which came out fine, they asked me to raise my knees up and then spread them as wide as possible. When I had them spread as wide as I could, I was told it was not enough. The pain in my hips was already agonizing, but I kept moving my knees apart with all the effort I could muster, making creaking sounds in the process till the technician was satisfied.

They took an exposure, and while they were gone to develop the film, I brought my knees together with a sigh of deliverance.

When they returned, they told me I had to take that one over again. Someone had walked into the dark room and turned on the lights while they were developing it. Getting repeat films for one reason or another was quite common in x-ray.

"That's a hell of a way to treat a patient," I said, and proceeded to go through the same ordeal again.

The next day the surgeon told me that another doctor had been studying my x-rays and felt that, rather than the "cups," the "total hip replacement" would be better for me. But nothing definite had yet been decided.

I learned later that the reason they were considering the total hip replacement was because my hip joints were in extremely bad condition.

A couple of days later the surgeon told me that, after a meeting, they were leaning heavily in favor of cups again.

Later, they scheduled the cups operation for the middle of the next week. They would do one hip, then, three months later, the other one.

After returning from a weekend pass, I was told by the surgeon that because of my rigid spine and the long bed rest the cups operation would be too much for me to bear. The results would be of small benefit to my ability to walk better than I already was walking with my short crutches, which was almost as fast as I used to walk.

The surgery I had dreaded was postponed indefinitely, and I was discharged from the hospital, with Stephanie and me in a happy and jovial mood.

At home, while Stephanie worked, I joyously resumed writing my novel with the companionship of a female Baltimore oriole that Stephanie had rescued after it had fallen out of its broken nest, with its eyes still closed and completely naked. The bird had grown to become a cheerful happy-go-lucky part of the family. It felt most comfortable perched on my shoulder or left hand that rested on my desk. It took naps with its beak buried in its feathery back, and occasionally it hopped onto my right hand to peck mischievously at my moving pencil. It frequently flew from my room to the kitchen for a bite to eat. Like people, it too had a personality of its own, albeit fortunately, a cheerful one.

We named it Gwendolyn, and for the year and a half that it lived with us, it gave us both a lot of pleasure. In the summer, we allowed it to fly into our big apple tree in the backyard where it happily trilled from branch to branch, eating insects. When we called to it, it would fly back to us and we'd bring it back into the house. When it finally decided to leave us, as we knew it would, it flew from the apple tree to a heavily wooded area beyond our yard and was gone forever. Stephanie wept.

Except for the occasional clinic visits I made at the hospital, that year was quite pleasant and in many ways joyous.

After I had completed the first draft of my novel, the medication I was taking for my arthritis caused my stomach to bleed again. Stephanie and I went to the hospital's emergency room, where I had a tube inserted into my nostril down to my stomach. With a syringe, a clear fluid was drawn from my stomach. The doctor said the bleeding was not in my upper stomach. My hematocrit (red blood count) indicated that I had lost a lot of blood. Therefore I had a needle inserted into a vein in my arm which was attached to an I.V. bottle on a pole.

After the doctor left, we waited for some time for an "escort" to take me to x-ray, then up to the Intensive Care Unit. In the meantime, Stephanie signed the admittance form and a nurse told us that hospital personnel had been reduced by five percent, mostly through attrition. The few new employees worked for lower wages.

When I finally got to the Medical Intensive Care Unit, I had wires attached to my chest to monitor my heartbeat and my nose tube was attached to a suction machine which kept my stomach clear of acids.

The next morning, I was sent to the x-ray department for an upper G.I. series. The x-rays proved negative. The doctors believed the bleeding, which had stopped, was caused by gastric irritation that was too small to show up on the film. I was then transferred to the ward for one day, and then discharged.

At home I resumed work on my novel, revising the first draft.

Gradually I resumed taking my medication till I was taking six Indocin and twenty aspirins per day. My arthritis was under fairly good control and everything seemed to be going well.

About six months later, however, my stools were not only again black as tar, but also covered with red blood. Stephanie drove me to the emergency room. I was again, for the third time, treated in the Intensive Care Unit, this time requiring a longer ice water treatment before the bleeding would stop. When it finally did, I was then transferred to the ward.

There the doctors, looking pleased, told me my hermatacrit had gone up almost to normal. They later told me I was doing very well and suggested that I consider getting the hip surgery now, rather than wait and have this recurrent stomach bleeding. They said I was in good shape and the hip surgery should benefit me so much that I could reduce my anti-inflammation medication drastically.

In the evening, Stephanie came to visit me, as she had been doing every day, and was surprised when she saw that I was not dressed in my street clothes. "I thought you said you would be discharged today," she said.

"I would've been. But I decided to get my hip surgery done."

"But your doctor told you to wait as long as possible, to give them a chance to perfect this operation," she admonished.

"Yeah I know, hon, but I already waited a long time since he told me that. Besides, the doctors think I should get the hips done now."

"Why now?" she asked.

"Because if I keep waiting, I'd have to keep taking large doses of Indocin and aspirins to keep the inflammation down. They're afraid that if I keep getting this stomach bleeding, they might not be able to stop it."

With her mouth slightly open, she held my gaze for a moment, then finally said, "Yes, I guess that makes sense."

As I waited for the surgery date to be settled, each passing day without my Indocin and aspirins made moving about increasingly more difficult and painful, even with my Canadian crutches, which I had received several months earlier.

Two doctors from the arthritis clinic came to see me and concluded that, at this point, the total hip replacement was my best bet. It looks like a unanimous decision, I thought. Nevertheless, I felt some trepidation.

The next day, Dr. R., an orthopedic surgeon, examined my legs. He had dark hair and was of average height. He told me he would need new x-rays and that I should get at least one week's therapy to build up my leg muscles before surgery.

Subsequently, after getting the x-rays, I was in Dr. R.'s office where Dr. R., Dr. G. and myself examined the x-rays and then discussed the surgery. Dr. R. said there were some risks, such as infection, but not really big ones. If an infection should occur in the hip prosthesis, then the prosthesis would have to be removed and I would have to walk without any hip joint. I would still be able to walk, he explained, but only for short distances.

This increased my trepidation for a moment, but it was quickly washed away by my indomitable optimism.

His partner, Dr. G., the quiet one and the actual surgeon of the team, added that the artificial hip joints would last for fifty years, according to tests. He did not mention how long the glue would last.

When I got back to the ward, Stephanie was already there waiting for me. After getting dressed, we left the hospital on a weekend pass.

A couple of days after returning to the hospital, Dr. R. told me my surgery would take place the following day. By now my hip joints felt like they were on fire, and I was anxious to get the surgery over with. But Dr. R. added that the surgery would only take place if the glue came in on time. There was a squabble at the hospital among the people there who "were protecting their own little empires," all claiming it was their province to order the glue. The result was that the glue had not been ordered. "We'll know by tonight whether the glue comes in."

"That's a hell of a way to run a railroad," I said.

"I agree with you," Dr. R. said. Then, extending his hands out from his sides and shrugging, he added, "But that, unfortunately, is the way things are."

In the evening, Dr. R. and Dr. G. returned to tell me that they had bad news for me. The glue had not come in, and the operation was postponed for two weeks.

Since I was all primed up for the surgery, I was terribly disappointed. "Oh, Christ!" I said to them. "Now I'll have to suffer two more weeks with these aching hips."

They cheered me up a bit when they offered to give me two weeks leave of absence.

But at home, without my medication, my hips were quite painful and, although I was happy to be home, I could not drive the car, ride the lawn mower, or put on my socks anymore.

When I got back to the hospital, I talked out in the hallway to a patient who had had one artificial hip put in and was waiting to get the other one done. He was a corncob-smoking, tall, bony man with a thick crop of white hair. A World War I veteran, he told me he was seventy-six years old and was very happy with his new hip joint. "It doesn't hurt me anymore," he said in his strong baritone voice. "But I gotta wait a while before they do the other one because I got blood clots."

Both of us were using Canadian crutches to walk with.

"Would you be able to discard those crutches after you get your other hip done?" I asked.

"Aw, sure I would," he said. "I don't need the crutches for my leg with the new hip. I kin stand on it like any rooster. It's the other hip that I need them for."

"Well, that sounds quite encouraging," I said.

"Let me tell ya', young fella, you'll never regret getting these new-fangled hip joints. They're the best thing that has come down the pike since God made little green apples."

After we had parted, I settled myself on my bed and rolled his words through my mind, especially the part about his feeling no more pain in that hip. I luxuriated over the realization that my poor aching hips had a lot to look forward to.

Dr. R. came in and told me the surgery would be done on one hip the following morning. Then I would have to wait four to six weeks after that before they would do the other hip. This would give my whole body a chance to recuperate from the major surgery.

An anesthesiologist interviewed me, wanting to know if I was allergic to anything. I said, "Not that I'm aware of."

He seemed satisfied, and said, "Well, everything checks out okay. We shouldn't have any problems." He got up from his chair, we shook hands and exchanged amenities, then he left with a contented expression on his face.

Later I had my right hip swabbed with Bethadine. Still later, with my crutches, I walked to the preparation room where I had my pubic, belly and thigh areas shaved. In the evening, I signed a consent form giving them permission to do the surgery.

On the day of the surgery, I got up at 6 A.M., moved my bowels, as I do every morning, washed up, then had my right hip again swabbed with Bethadine. An hour later, a nurse had me remove my clean pajamas under my bed covers, then she gave me two injections in the left hip. A few minutes later, a stretcher arrived and I was wheeled into the operating room. A nurse in a green gown, mask and cap, asked me some questions, including one on whether I was taking steroids. I told her that I had, but not lately. I asked her why she wanted to know that. She said that if I was still taking steroids, they would have to give me some because my body would need them during anesthesia.

There were three other masked bandits in the room, whom I could not identify. I was pretty well tranquilized by then, and did not very much care who they were. I was transferred from the stretcher to the operating table. A needle was inserted into a vein of my left arm for fluid intake, another nurse stuck a needle into my right arm, then one near my left breast, and immediately I felt groggy and soon lost consciousness.

I was brought back to consciousness by a terrible choking pain in my throat. I could not breathe. Something blunt was pushing itself into my throat causing me to cough, which I was unable to do. I was gasping for air, actually being strangled to death by something or someone.

I managed to open my eyes to see one of the masked persons up on the table, trying like a madman to push something down my throat. At the same time I heard someone say, "All right, you can stop it now."

The masked person suddenly relaxed his pressure, removed the breathing tube from the entrance of my throat and I was gloriously able to breathe again. Immediately after that, I dozed off.

I was awakened by a nurse in the recovery room. The first thing I said was, "How did the operation go?" She looked at me sympathetically, and said, "They did not do it."

I was stunned and was barely able to mumble my disappointment when Dr. R. came in. He explained to me that, because they could not get my arthritic neck back, they could not get the breathing tube down my throat. Therefore they had to cancel the hip surgery.

Later, an ear, nose and throat doctor came to see me. He was a hawk-nosed, nervous, chain-smoking little man who told me that the only way they could get a breathing tube into my windpipe would be through a tracheotomy. This required making an incision into my throat which the doctor assured me would not be too bad.

After a while, I was wheeled back to my ward, wondering why these learned doctors did not anticipate the breathing tube problem before I went to the operating room and before I was anesthetized. This was the second time I almost received my surgery. The first was when the glue was not ordered on time. This incredible, on-and-off-again surgery left a bitter taste of resentment in my mouth.

One of the three other patients in the room, R., a black man who had a "cup" put in his hip several weeks ago and was still bed-ridden, said, "How'd it go, Mike?" "It didn't go," I told him. Then I explained why and ended with an angry, "I don't think these people in this hospital know what the hell they're doing."

"Oh, they know what they're doin'," R. said. "They sometime have their bad days too. You watch, they will come up with a way to do it."

As soon as Dr. R. came to talk to me about alternatives, my anger dissipated like a drop of water on a hot stove. I eagerly listened as he explained the two options they had, either a spinal or the incision into my throat. But there were two drawbacks to the spinal. The first was that it might not work on my rigid spine, and the second was that it would last for only a limited time, which would bode badly for me if my feeling came back while the surgery was still in progress.

These last words sent a frightening chill up my spine. It was clear to me that Dr. R. was leaning toward the tracheotomy. Then he added, "With the tracheotomy you would be completely under and the machine would breathe for you if you needed it." I did not care for any of the options, but the tracheotomy seemed the safest.

"Which one do you recommend?" I asked.

"Frankly," Dr. R. said slowly, "I think the tracheotomy would give us better control." We finally settled on the tracheotomy. Then Dr. R. said, "Next Thursday, two days from now, we will try again. But this time we will try to do both hips in that one operation, because we wouldn't want to put you through two tracheotomies unless it was absolutely necessary. But, I want to emphasize, we will do it only if everything goes well."

I was very pleased with the idea of having both hips done at once, rather than having to go through surgery twice.

The next morning, Dr. R. told me they had decided that their best bet was to give me the spinal with a tube so they could keep injecting the anesthesia for as long as was necessary. I was a bit disconcerted by all this back-and-forth switching, but I saw no reason to protest their decision and went along with it.

After breakfast, I took a shower, then sat in my chair to do some reading. A small Oriental anesthesiologist came to talk to me. He was a pleasant, soft-spoken person with a friendly smile. He said he did not like the spinal because it would not give him full control over my vital organs. Besides that, it would be very uncomfortable for me, and it also might not be possible to get a tap into my spine. He felt it would be best to try to get a tube through my nose into the windpipe. If that failed, then a tracheotomy would be the next best thing to do.

After he left, I felt that he was the only one so far who made sense. He seemed to be fully experienced and seemed to know precisely what had to be done and what approach would be best for the patient. It was perceptible to me that the surgeons were making their decisions in secret chambers without the participation of all the operating room members.

The right hand did not seem to know what the left hand was doing. I crossed my fingers and hoped they would get their act together before I went to surgery on the following morning.

Later, the hawk-nosed, chain-smoking doctor came in to examine my throat, and announced that there was plenty of room for a tracheotomy.

A nurse brought me a form to sign giving the surgeons permission to do the bilateral hip replacements and a tracheotomy.

In the evening, after visiting hours, a nurse gave me three enemas, two aspirins, a valium and an antibiotic. Everything was all set for the next morning's surgery. I was confident that everything would be under control and, regardless of what the operation entailed, I was willing to withstand it so that soon I would be able to walk again without pain and without crutches.

Despite the tranquilizer I had taken, I found it impossible to fall asleep. My mind was too excited and rambled freely.

I recalled how I had met Stephanie at a dance ballroom where the big-name bands played. I was attracted by her slim loveliness and her sense of humor. We saw each other almost every day and soon got married.

I was driving tractor-trailers at that time and Stephanie

went with me on many trips. We both worked and bought a home in Mullins and we were both delighted when she became pregnant. But a few weeks later, she developed severe cramps. I phoned her gynecologist, who told me to get her to the hospital immediately. Her pain was so bad she could hardly walk without my support. When I got her to the hospital her blood pressure was very low and the doctor would not operate till they could get it back up. In the bed she twisted, moaned and screamed as she hemorrhaged internally while I watched in frustrating helplessness. In the evening the nurse urged me to leave.

With Stephanie's pain-racked face embedded in my vision, I drove home almost in a trance and, despite being brought up in John Wayne's world where men never cry, I let the tears roll down my cheeks in hot rivers of remorse and anguish.

The following morning when I got to the hospital, I learned that she was still in the operating room. I waited for a long time before she was brought out. She looked more dead than alive, but they assured me that she would be all right.

Her doctor told me she would have had twins but the fetuses were stuck in the falopian tubes, which had become ruptured. The fetuses were removed, her fallopian tubes had to be tied off, and she would never again be able to have any children, which made us both very sad.

Stephanie went through a period of deep depression, then she recovered fully.

At this point, the tranquilizer finally put me to sleep.

Early in the morning I was awakened by a nurse, given two more injections, then I was wheeled on a stretcher to the operating room.

I was at last on the threshold of getting new hips, and I saw vivid images of my being able to walk again without crutches or pain. As far as I was concerned, to accomplish such a miracle, the surgical ordeal would be a small price to pay.

With hypnotic fascination I watched one of the masked doctors inject Lydicaine under the skin of my throat. Then, with a scalpel, he painlessly slit the skin and the windpipe and inserted a black plastic breathing tube, and I immediately lost consciousness.

Chapter 2

On waking up in the recovery room, I was told by a nurse that both hips had been done. Unable to speak because of the tracheotomy in my throat, I responded with a gigantic smile.

I was moved to the post-operative ward, which contained about a half dozen beds where everything appeared to me as hazy and dream-like. Thirst was my most acute sensation, and only a few sips of water were all I was allowed.

Stephanie was there at my bedside, her face looking tired and grim. I squeezed her hand and smiled, and she smiled back. Though she had heard the nurses' assurances that I was all right, she now knew from me for certain that this was indeed so.

Dr. R. came in greeting us with a cautious smile, after which his expression became serious as he turned his attention to the breathing tube attached to my tracheotomy; he adjusted the oxygen flow to a specific pressure and mixed it with a specific saline mist.

With that done, his smile returned with more certainty

and he said to Stephanie, "Your husband surprised everyone in the operating room. Even though he had lost a lot of blood he had more stamina than all of us put together."

Dr. R. had already related that to me in the operating recovery room and I was delighted to see Stephanie laugh at this news.

Then she said, "I believe you, Dr. R., he often surprises me too."

I was confident that I would hold up my end of the surgical ordeal, but I was not very certain that the medical staff would hold up their end. Since I was obsessed with staying alive, I kept myself alert around the clock, waking up to watch the nurses' every move. Whenever they came to my bedside to take my vital signs, adjust the oxygen flow or change the I.V. bottles, I would observe every detail with a critical eye.

For instance, every time the I.V. bottles were changed, I always watched for air bubbles in the line leading into my vein. Whenever I saw bubbles, I would bring it to the nurse's attention and she would simply disconnect the tubing and drain it till all the bubbles were gone.

One nurse, however, who had made the bottle change, did only a cursory drainage, leaving high up in the line a long air bubble, and started walking away. I quickly signaled her back and, with my hand, I pinched the tube to stop the fluid flow. With my other hand, I pointed to the bubble.

She told me that the bubble was not too large and it would dissolve in my blood stream without causing me any harm. When I refused to release the tubing, she became peeved but soon relented, disconnected the tubing and drained out the air bubble. I was satisfied.

Later, one of the night nurses had asked me if I ever slept. Every time she came to my bed, she would find me lying there with my eyes open. I was surprised by this news because I was sure that I was getting my sleep and I assumed that it was just that I would open my eyes the moment I sensed someone by my bed. It was not till some days later that I was told by other nurses, including Stephanie, that I slept with my eyes open. I guess my newly developed paranoia has created all kinds of wonders, I said to myself.

When I woke up in the morning, I became horror-stricken when I saw that my hands and arms had turned pale yellow and the veins looked like bright yellow snakes.

Frantically I waved my arms to attract a nurse. A nurse arrived immediately and looked at my arms, and her placid expression turned grim. Then she blurted, "I'll call Dr. R."

Dr. R. was there within minutes. He examined my arms, chest and face, and with a worried expression told me that my liver was being overworked. He explained that I had lost a large amount of blood in the operating room and that the liver was now engaged in the enormous task of cleaning out the dead blood cells which had resulted from the many transfusions I had received.

"What can you do for it?" I asked.

"Nothing. We just have to let it run its course."

After he left with an unhappy expression on his face, I felt like a passenger on a sinking ship whose captain and crew had just rowed away in a lifeboat.

Having had a rudimentary knowledge of hepatitis, I knew that what I had was hepatitis, regardless of what had caused it. It had to run its course through its victims, killing some and sparing some. You win some and you lose some, I thought. Anyway since it was not 100 percent fatal, I surmised that, simply because I wanted to live, I would be among those who would fully recover.

The tall, lean and silent Dr. G. suddenly appeared at my bedside. Without saying a word to me he examined my yellow skin with a frowning expression on his face. A minute or so later, he turned and went out as silently as he had come in.

Since I had come out of the operating room I had been and still was disconnecting my breathing tube from my tracheotomy to cough up phlegm into tissue paper which I discarded into a paper bag taped to the bed railing. This I did every half hour or so, day and night, whenever the tracheotomy would clog up.

It was in the middle of one of these coughing sessions that Dr. R. returned to my bedside. When I stopped coughing, he listened to my heart with his stethoscope and said, "You're doing fine." I nodded with a grin and in sign language I tried to convey to him, "I know that."

"You can talk, you know," he said. "Just disconnect the tube and hold your hand over the trach."

I did not think it was possible to talk with the tube in my throat, but I tried it anyway. My first effort proved futile, then I heard myself say, "I can't do it." Because I was doing what I said I could not do, it made us both burst out in laughter.

From then on, talking was easy as long as I held my hand tightly over the opening and kept the tracheotomy clear of phlegm.

After Stephanie got out of work, she ate supper, then came to visit me, and her smiling face immediately reverted to a look of horror. "Oh, my God!" were her first words. "What happened to your face? It's...it's all yellow!"

I smiled at her as I unhooked the tracheotomy, coughed to clear out the phlegm, then put my hand over the opening, and said, "It's nothing, hon. It was caused by all the transfusions I had. It'll clear up as soon as my liver clears out all the dead blood cells."

Her expression now turned to one of amazement, and she said, "You're able to talk! How on earth did you do that?"

After I had explained it to her, she then said, "What was that about dead cells?" After I repeated it to her, she asked, "What kind of dead cells?"

"The cells that were killed when the stored blood was frozen."

"But a lot of people get transfusions," she said. "But they never turn yellow."

"Remember when I had my stomach bleedings? I got only a couple of units of blood at a time and there were not that many dead blood cells to cause me to turn yellow. But the hip operation lasted eight hours and I lost all of my blood and it all had to be replaced with stored blood. You see the difference?"

She paused a moment, then said, "Yes, I think I do."

On the third day after surgery, Dr. R. took the plastic tube out of my throat and taped a four-by-four bandage over the opening. When I tried to speak, I still had to hold my hand over the throat opening to keep the air from escaping.

On the fourth day, I was alarmed when I woke up in the morning to find the skin around my throat, shoulders and upper chest covered with massive balloon-like swellings. The swellings were cushion soft and when pressed, they crackled like breakfast cereal. Hideous as these large swollen pouches were, my yellow skin gave them an even more bizarre appearance.

I called the nurse over, she felt the crackling swellings, and told me she had never seen anything like that before. Then she got on the phone and called Dr. R.

Dr. R. soon arrived, probed the swellings, then said, "That's all air under there. Every time you held your hand over the opening to cough or to talk, you pushed more and more air under your skin."

A short while after Dr. R. had left, the small, nervous ear, nose and throat doctor came in with a very harried expression on his face. He fingered the air cushions, his large eyes buggered out with worry, and with a frown said, "Dr. R. shouldn't have taken that tube out. If the air had reached your heart, you could've died of embolism."

With a small camera and a flash bulb, he took a couple of photos of the swollen areas. After that he put another plastic tube into my throat opening, hooked it up to the long flexible tube and adjusted the oxygen and saline mist flow, then he left.

The possible embolism that I so feared from the I.V. lines had unexpectedly crept into my body via another route. One hand not knowing what the other hand was doing was tantamount to me being surrounded by assassins, I thought with a shudder.

Nevertheless, with the breathing tube back in my throat, a certain sense of security returned to me. A day or two later, the air was completely gone from under my skin, but the yellow tinge still remained. All my nights since the surgery had been filled with constant pain from my hips, but they were gradually getting less painful.

However, the heels of my feet, which were propped up with sandbags to keep the toes pointing toward the ceiling, felt as though they were resting on hot charcoals. My stomach was bloated with air from the oxygen and it was difficult to pass the gas, which caused me much discomfort. This discomfort made talking even more uncomfortable, leaving me to speak only when it was absolutely necessary.

Within a few days, the yellow tinge in my skin was discernibly fading, to Dr. R.'s and my great consolation. This indicated that my liver had survived the task of clearing out of my bloodstream all the dead cells.

Dr. R. told me that, although I was feeling miserable, I was doing remarkably well, and that I was ready to be moved to the ward.

In the afternoon, two nurses arrived from the ward, disconnected my breathing tube from the oxygen and the saline mist, and moved me, bed and all, out of Intensive Care to the elevator—where there was the usual long wait—then finally up to the fourth floor and into a four-patient room.

The head nurse, a tiny, nervous woman of middle age with jet black hair, supervised the project of getting me settled. She and another nurse expended an inordinately long time figuring out the mysterious mechanics of putting up a trapeze over the bed and a pair of pulleys at the foot for my leg exercises.

In the meantime, in an effort to advise them, I discovered that I was no longer able to speak. Without the oxygen and the saline mist, the tracheotomy had dried up, making it impossible for me to cough to clear it out, leaving me with only my nose to breathe through.

When the two nurses had finished putting up the trapeze and the pulleys, they turned their attention to the oxygen and mist controls. After much fumbling, they tried to hook the hose to my breathing tube. Seeing that the vapors coming out of the hose were very weak, I protested by putting one hand over my throat tube and, with the other hand, waving away the hose.

The head nurse, assuming that I was just being obstinate, told me in no uncertain terms that I had to have it hooked up. Full of frustration at my inability to speak, I signaled her for a pencil and paper. The other nurse handed me a pencil and pad and I wrote on it that the water vapor was too weak. The head nurse read it, then sarcastically told me that she knew what she was doing. "The doctor has ordered forty percent oxygen and that is what I'm giving you," she insisted.

Having spent days in the post-operative unit with the breathing tube, I knew that the oxygen and the water vapors had come out of the hose in a thick solid stream, and that what she was giving me was obviously not right.

Frantically, I wrote another note, this time handing it to

the other nurse requesting her to get Dr. R. or get me back downstairs so I could properly breathe again.

When Dr. R. arrived, I wrote him a note telling him that my throat tube was clogged and that the oxygen and vapor were not correct. Dr. R. removed the plastic tube from my throat, inserted a new one, then set the oxygen and the saline vapor to their correct strong pressure flow, and the issue was settled to my satisfaction.

With pain-killing drugs and a sleeping pill, I slept through the night with very little difficulty. If I had allowed the head nurse to hook me up to a weak vapor flow, I believe that from my sleep I would have never again awakened.

My days continued to be filled with stomach discomfort. In the mornings, I would have a good appetite, but by late afternoon, I could barely eat anything because my stomach would become too bloated with gas that refused to be passed. This great discomfort made me bad company for Stephanie and other visitors, such as relatives and friends, and it would continue for as long as I had the tube in my throat.

At last, Dr. R. removed the I.V. from the vein in my arm. Then he removed the breathing tube from my throat and placed a bandage over it. To speak, I still had to hold my hand over it, but this time the skin around the incision was healed, and there was no longer any danger of getting air under the skin again. Gradually, the slit in my throat would get smaller till it healed completely.

Shortly after that, Dr. R. and Dr. G. neared the end of their residency and another team of orthopedic surgeons arrived to get acquainted with the patients and their medical records.

One of these new doctors, Dr. B., introduced himself, then he removed the bandages from both my hips, leaving the stitches in place for later extraction.

He told me that my hematocrit had gone up to 25, and I

was allowed to sit up for a few minutes at a time. At first I felt a bit whoozy, but I soon became acclimated to the sitting position and felt fine. Also, my hips no longer ached me.

Later, with a sling and a hydraulic crane, I was lifted out of bed and lowered into a cushioned recliner chair with wheels. Stephanie pushed me along the hallway, stopping for a while at a large window to admire the outside world, then ending in the recreation room. But after about an hour of sitting in the chair, I felt a lot of discomfort under my right thigh near the hip joint. Stephanie pushed me back to my room and, with the crane, I was put back into bed.

This was the first hint that there was something wrong with my artificial hip joint, but because the doctors had assured me that everything had gone well in surgery, I assumed that it was nothing more than a muscle spasm.

At bedtime my right hip again acted up, this time with considerably more pain. I put my call light on and the night nurse, a sensitive former Navy nurse, came into the room. I asked her to set up the pulleys so that I could do some leg exercises to try to relieve the hip pain. But the exercises only aggravated the pain and suddenly the back of my thigh muscle cramped up into an excruciating knot. I again called for the nurse. When she arrived she did not know what to do for me, so she gave me a valium.

After an hour of no relief from the valium, I called her for the third time and she massaged my thigh, which felt as if it had steel cables running through it. The massaging helped very little and she was distressed by her inability to relieve my suffering. She called Dr. B. at his home and woke him from his sleep. Nurses do not call doctors at home except in emergencies. The doctor told her that it was probably nothing more than a bad muscle spasm and advised her to put a hot damp compress on it.

She put the compress around my thigh, sat me up on the

34 FOOTSTEPS TO SURVIVAL

edge of the bed, and put my feet in a pan of warm water. Soon the spasm was gone. She then helped me lay back in the bed, and the sudden freedom from the terrible pain enveloped me in a beautiful euphoria that drifted me into a deep sleep.

The next morning, I was again lifted out of bed by the crane and placed in the wheelchair. A pretty Red Cross volunteer named Julia pushed me along the hallways, stopping now and then to look out the windows and to chat a while.

At night, since I had had to keep my toes pointed toward the ceiling to guard against "frog legs," the heels of my feet had become quite raw and burned incessantly, making sleep virtually impossible.

In the morning, after breakfast, I was put on a stretcher and sent to Physical Therapy. A young woman therapist gently manipulated my legs to slowly increase their range of motion. After that she gave me two five-pound weights with which to strengthen my arms to enable me to begin walking with Canadian crutches.

When I got back to my room, Dr. B. and his pipe-smoking partner, Dr. A., removed the stitches from both my hips. Then Dr. B. examined my throat incision and said it had healed and that my stomach bloating should begin to subside. He also stopped the antibiotics I had been getting since my surgery.

At supper time, I was surprised at how easily my stomach accepted food, and there was no longer any bloating. When Stephanie arrived in the evening she commmented on how well and alert I looked.

At my next therapy session, I relished the fact that I would be walking on crutches, and eventually without them. The young woman therapist placed my wheelchair at one end of a pair of waist-high parallel bars, locked the wheels, and then asked me to stand up. I pushed myself up and was delighted at how smoothly and painlessly my new hip joints worked, free of the old noisy creakings. I then put my hands on the parallel bars and she told me to just stand like that for a while to get used to the standing position. I felt quite comfortable standing up, and when she told me to start walking between the parallel bars with my arms bearing much of the weight, I did so with child-like eagerness.

"Hold it! Hold it! Not too fast!" she called with a smile. "Now turn around and walk back slowly."

I had walked about fifteen feet, then slowly walked back to the wheelchair, where she told me to sit and take a short rest. Although I did not feel tired, I rested anyway. After that I got up and walked the full length of the parallel bars, which were about thirty feet long, then back to the wheelchair for another rest. All I felt was a slight weakness in my legs. "You did that very well," she said.

After being returned to my room, I ate dinner sitting in the wheelchair, then felt a slight tiredness drop over me and was ready for the bed. This time I needed the help of just one nurse. I stood up by myself and sat on the edge of the bed. Then, as I layed back, the nurse helped lift my legs up onto the bed and I slept soundly for nearly an hour.

Back in therapy on the following morning, I had my legs exercised on the table. Then I walked between the parallel bars, astonished at how firm my legs felt, and I walked back and forth along the full length of the bars four or five times without stopping. I felt no pain and would have walked longer had the therapist not stopped me.

The next day in therapy, after doing my leg exercises, I walked between the parallel bars using Canadian crutches for support. After that I walked a couple of laps around the therapy room with the therapist walking behind me holding my hips in the event I should lose my balance. I wanted to continue walking, but she told me it was enough for now.

After dinner, I walked with my crutches a little in the ward. In the evening when Stephanie was there, I walked with her along the hallway to her great delight.

I again brought the hard lump on the back of my thigh to the doctor's attention. He examined it and still insisted that it was a bunched-up muscle. I told him that I was not able to sleep on my right side because it hurt me too much to lay on the lump. He assured me that eventually it would not bother me. Although I was beginning to have my doubts about his explanation, I nevertheless hoped he was right.

He then examined my left hip and removed some stitches that the show-off Dr. A. had overlooked.

They had no plans for letting me go so soon on a weekend pass, but I managed to convince him that it was essential to my well-being, so he reluctantly gave me one.

After calling Stephanie, I got dressed in my street clothes, then when she arrived we left immediately, saying goodbye to the patients and the nurses. Stephanie pushed me in a wheelchair down to the lobby. Then I got out of the chair and with my crutches walked to the car—and had no trouble getting in—after which she drove us home.

At home, I was amazed at how easily I was able to climb the back porch steps, although Stephanie was behind me just in case. Stephanie was very happy to have me back home, even though it would be for only Saturday and Sunday.

On the first day, I had an opportunity to write my every-two-weeks newspaper column titled "Brass Tacks." I had been writing the labor column for *Modern Times*, a left-leaning anti-war newspaper in New Haven, for the past few months. Since I was always way ahead of my schedule with my material, I had never missed a single deadline despite my lengthy hospital stay.

My brother Bill came to our home in the afternoon to see how I was doing. He was quite surprised when he had gone to the hospital to visit me to learn that I had already left on a weekend pass.

Back in the hospital, I was in Physical Therapy at 10 A.M., where I was lowered by a hoist into the big Hubbard tub of swirling warm water. I did my leg exercises, and the therapist left. I was wearing a bathing suit and felt like a kid again swimming in a running stream and diving from rocky cliffs into deep pools of water.

I felt an affinity with the primeval urges of our past when all life began. Whether it was the fresh water streams of Connecticut or the salt waters of the Long Island Sound, I enjoyed nothing better than to immerse myself in these fluid revitalizers. During the summer months when school was out and between various jobs, my brother Joe and I often fished in Long Island Sound with some friends. When we tired of fishing, we would dive from the rowboat and swim in our vast but long-forgotten aquatic cradle, enjoying ourselves immensely.

As I soaked in the swirling water of the Hubbard tub, I sensed myself smiling at these old memories. Then I wondered why we all had to grow up and lose our healthy spontaneity.

In the afternoon, Dr. R. came into my room to see me walk on crutches. I took them up and walked out of the room and he followed me. Then he asked me to walk down the hallway, which I did at a fairly fast pace.

Dr. R. chased after me, saying, "Hold it, I'm not a young man!"

I slowed down and said, "What's the matter, friend, can't you keep up?"

He laughed. "You've progressed faster than we had estimated."

"Of course I did." I laughed. "That's because I'm trying to get away from all of you doctors."

I then changed the subject and asked him to feel the hard lump on my right thigh. After he felt it, he too said it was nothing more than a lumped-up muscle.

Later, Dr. B. told me my hermatacrit had gone up to almost normal and that I would be discharged from the hospital the next week. But I would still have to continue going to Physical Therapy. I told him my wife worked every day and I had no transportation. He then thought it would be best if I remained in the hospital for at least three more weeks of therapy. Although I preferred being at home, under the circumstances I acquiesed to his suggestion.

As the days passed, I found myself doing things that prior to surgery I was unable to do. I was by then capable of climbing in and out of the Hubbard tub all by myself, and could peddle the stationary bicycle with speed and ease. My therapist remarked that I was doing very well.

Back in the ward, Dr. R. came to see me with a camera and flash bulbs and asked me to come out to the recreation room so he could take a couple of full-length photographs of me. (He already had taken a set of them prior to surgery.)

As we entered the empty recreation room, Dr. R. said, "You know, you made history in this hospital."

"Oh yeah, what'd I do now?"

"You're the first patient to ever have two total hip replacements done in one surgery."

With my crutches I stood beside the pool table and he snapped a front view and side view of me.

Later, when we compared the "before and after" photos, we saw a dramatic difference. The first set showed me bent over almost doubled up at the waist and looking drawn and worn out, despite the smile on my face. The second set showed me standing ramrod straight with a healthy, smiling pink face that looked ten years younger than the first.

Dr. B. ordered a new set of hip X-rays, which had to be

duplicated because the first set had not developed properly. From my own experience, I had found that it was commonplace to be exposed to extra X-rays due to technicians' carelessness, and what made it even worse was that there was no system for monitoring patient exposure to dangerous X-ray radiation. X-rays were ordered arbitrarily by practically every doctor involved with a patient, putting the patient's life in jeopardy.

Back in my room, I sat on the edge of my bed conversing with one of the patients when Dr. A. came in. I asked him about my X-rays. He told me that there was a slight abnormality in my right prosthesis. Rather than elaborate on it, he simply said that Dr. B. would talk to me about it and he left the room.

When my supper tray arrived, I had suddenly lost my appetite. I was stunned and sat there in a daze chewing listlessly on my food and not even tasting it. The knot in my thigh and the abnormal prosthesis X-ray swirled through my mind. I had the frightening conviction that there was something very seriously wrong with that hip joint.

It was bad enough to have this information dropped on me so suddenly by that heartless, pipe-smoking Dr. A., but to keep me in suspense was the sharpest cut of all. It is the unknown that frightens us the most, and if he had only told me precisely what the abnormality was, I would have been able to face up to it and begin plotting a way to circumvent it the way I have always done in my long fight for survival.

When Stephanie came to pick me up for my weekend pass, I stopped eating and we left the room. On our way to the elevator, we met Dr. B. in the hallway and I asked him for details about my hip abnormality. He invited Stephanie and me into his office. Dr. A. was there sitting at one of the two desks, reading a chart and leisurely smoking his pipe, suggesting a smug, country club ambiance.

Dr. B. showed us the right hip X-rays. The front view showed the stainless steel spike, which was attached to the femur ball, correctly placed down inside the center of the femur bone. But the side view showed the spike protruding about three quarters of an inch out of the bone, and I instantly realized that the surgeons, Dr. R. and Dr. G., had botched it up. For a moment, both anger and helplessness welled up in me.

"How on earth did that happen?" I said.

Dr. B. explained that the spike had broken through the bone which was too weak from lack of exercise. By exercising, the bone might become stronger and it could heal in that position and nothing need be done. On the other hand, too much exercise could aggravate it.

My instincts told me that he was full of feces, but my ignorance subdued me, and I said to myself, "Who am I to challenge the learned doctor?" When we left his office, I was devastated.

As Stephanie drove us home, we both remained silent for a while, then she said, "I don't understand how that thing could break through your bone like that."

"I don't understand it either," I said.

We both fell into another silence. I just sat there running it all through my mind, carefully examining every event that had taken place since the surgery trying to fathom this strange phenomenon. I could not comprehend how it was possible for the spike to erode through the bone without my feeling it. It just did not make sense to me. Finally, I concluded that my instincts were indeed correct and that Dr. B.'s opinion was nothing more than a wild guess, the same as his diagnosis that the spike was only a hard muscle knot.

To me, the most logical explanation was that the prosthesis had been put in at that abnormal angle during the surgery and the reason it was not detected earlier was because the post-operative X-rays were only of the front view, where the abnormality was not visible. By the time we got home, I had regained my equilibrium and my spirits rose, bringing me back to my old optimistic self again.

At home, I told Stephanie my theory and her expression immediately brightened.

"That sure makes more sense than Dr. B. did," she said. "Does that spike bother you?"

"No, my thigh muscles are getting used to it."

"But you won't be able to sleep on your right side anymore," she said.

"I'll live with it," I said, trying to console both of us. "Things could have been worse."

Yet, as I wondered whether the abnormality would cause me problems later, a residue of uneasiness haunted the outer edges of my optimism.

I went to my room and sat in my swivel chair at my desk and busied myself in the creative world of writing. This was my sanctuary where all the "slings and arrows of outrageous fortune" could not touch me.

Here, I pondered the whats, wheres and whys of life, the earth, moon, sun, galaxies, black holes and the wonders of the entire universe, becoming ecstatic over inspiring discoveries that helped the mind to grow and conquer any adversity.

Chapter 3

When my weekend pass ended, Stephanie and I left for the hospital. This time I drove the car, which was the first time since surgery, and I drove it with ease and perfect control.
Dr. B. asked me if I had been worried over the weekend.
"I wasn't worried," I said. "After reviewing it in my mind I came to the conclusion that the prosthesis did not erode through the bone, but had been installed in that awkward position during surgery."
He smiled and said, "I had also reached the same conclusion."
In the afternoon, I was sent to X-ray, where I received lamigram X-rays of my right hip. The lamigram consisted of a series of X-rays taken at different depths. A certain amount of worry settled over me as I wondered what it was they were looking for.
The next morning, I asked Dr. B. if he had seen the lamination X-rays. He said he had not seen them yet, but was quite certain the prosthesis was stable. It was just that Dr. A. wanted these X-rays done. I was seized by a sudden anger. That pipe-smoking, son-of-a-bitch Dr. A. had not only put

me through a lot of mental anguish, but had also exposed me to a lot of X-ray radiation that was absolutely unnecessary. All of which was done, it seemed to me, to puff up his mediocre importance.

Later, Dr. B. told me he had seen the X-rays and the abnormal prosthesis was indeed stable. I asked him about the glue, whether it had been pushed through the hole in the bone and could possibly be floating around somewhere in my flesh. He assured me that it did not go through, the glue was put only partially into the hole. I was greatly palliated to hear this.

When I finally received my discharge, I phoned Stephanie the good news, then I went to the nurses' station where the secretary made my clinic appointment.

Dr. B. came by and informed me that he had told Dr. R. about the abnormality in my right hip and Dr. R. was flabbergasted. Then Dr. B. added that I had made a remarkable recovery and that he wished all patients were like me.

Back in my room, I got dressed. Stephanie arrived, and we said goodbye to the other patients in the room. Then we left. One of the nurses who had been taking care of me came along with us as far as the lobby, wished me good luck and kissed me on the cheek. Then Stephanie and I got into the car and I drove us home. We were both happy that I was finally out of the hospital, not very much worse for the wear.

On my first Orthopedic Clinic appointment day, Stephanie stayed home from work to go with me. Since the clinic was crowded as usual, we knew we would have a very long wait. We checked in to establish our place, then went up to the fourth floor to visit some of the patients and nurses I had befriended.

After nearly an hour, we returned to the clinic where we still had another hour or two to wait. There we met J., a young Viet Nam veteran with stomach ulcers who had shared my room briefly and who was hostile to and uncooperative with the doctors and nurses. He did pushups day or night whenever his stomach bothered him. He was in a wheelchair, his light brown hair was in a tangle and he looked pale, haggard, and very ill. He told me he was not feeling good. Later he was wheeled away to admittance.

We then met T., the black man who had a cup put into his hip. He told me he was having all kinds of problems with it and it was causing him a lot of pain. Then I met the carpenter who was still having trouble with his shoulder despite the surgery he had had on it.

J. was also there, but he said he was getting along fine with the plate in his hip.

When my name was finally called, I went into one of the examining rooms. Dr. B. and Dr. A. examined me briefly and were very pleased at how well I looked. Then they told me that Dr. R. also wanted to see me.

After a short wait, Dr. R. called me into his room. He showed me the X-rays with the spike at an angle and expressed his sorrow over it. He said that if the part of the spike that was sticking out of the bone should bother me, they could easily saw it off. I told him that it only bothered me if I slept on my right side which I did not do any more.

Also there was some discomfort when I climbed stairs and the thigh muscle crossed over the sharp spike tip. He told me that the muscle would eventually develop a bursa, a hard covering that would allow the muscle to slide over the spike with no discomfort. He also added that, if there should be a need to put the spike in straight, which there was no need for now, the spike could be pulled out without too much difficulty. The glue had a strong compression strength, but not a very strong tension strength. He compared it to a cement block, but with much finer granules.

He wanted to see how well I walked without my crutches,

which I was able to do for short distances, and he was pleased by how well I did it. But he suggested I stay with the crutches a while longer.

Then he had me stand on one leg at a time, which I did with ease. After that, he checked my posture. Then he had me lie down on the table where he checked the range of motion in both legs. He then recorded it.

"Your leg ranges are very good," he said. "I suggest that you do a few more abduction exercises."

I had been doing all my other leg exercises except the abductions. "Okay, I'll do a few more of them," I said.

"They're very necessary to walking," he added.

My next appointment was for the arthritis clinic. After getting weighed, I sat with Stephanie in the crowded waiting area. Dr. C., who had been following up my problems from the beginning, saw me sitting in the hallway and asked me if I would not mind having two student nurses interview me for a report they needed. I told him I did not mind. He introduced me to the two young ladies and we made an appointment for them to come to my home on the following Thursday morning.

When I was finally called into the examining room, the two student nurses went in with me. (They already had permission from Dr. C. and myself.)

In the room there was a young doctor still in training. After I had been introduced to him, Dr. C. asked him to diagnose my problem. I put my crutches in the corner, walked to the center of the room and stood as straight as I could. After a moment the doctor said, "Ankylosing Spondylitis."

Dr. C. looked at me and said, "Should we give him an 'A' for that?"

"Sure, why not, he did good," I said.

Then Dr. C. asked me a number of routine questions,

which I answered while the other doctor and the two young nurses listened.

Then I told him about my knees, which were often sore and swollen. He said increased activity had caused them to swell, but that aspirin and rest should keep the swelling down. However, if it continued giving me trouble, then steroid injections would help. I mentioned that I was worried that my knees would become a big problem. He did not feel that they would. The problem could be controlled by exercising the knees to maintain the range of motion.

On Thursday, the two student nurses, who were from the University of Bridgeport, came to my home to interview me. They asked me how the arthritis began and how it affected me.

I told them that the first symptoms began when I was in my early thirties and driving tractor-trailers, which often involved loading and unloading heavy freight. One night, after three years of that, I experienced severe pains in my upper back that forced me out of bed to seek relief by walking around the kitchen.

For the first couple of days the pain did not return. Then when it did, it returned almost every night thereafter.

It was at this point that I decided to quit driving and returned to my tool-and-die-making trade, and for several years I worked without any physical problems.

But when I quit the factory I had worked at to work for more money in an air-conditioned plant where highly precisioned instruments were manufactured, I began to become afflicted with attacks of stiff neck that at first would come and go. But then they began to retain their grip for longer periods, till the vertebrae in my neck had become fused together and I could no longer turn my head in either direction.

The two student nurses were taking notes and encouraged

me to go on, so I told them that slowly over the years the pain and inflammation worked their way down my spine. I then went to a doctor who told me that it was nothing more than strained muscles due to overexertion. Because my job was no longer strenuous, I did not believe the doctor, and I did not see any point in seeing other doctors.

I learned to live with the pain, alleviating much of it by eating aspirin as though it was candy. By that time, it had become obvious to me that I was a victim of arthritis. My mother and father and brothers and sister had no joint problems, neither did any of my other blood relatives. (I later learned from Dr. C. that it nevertheless was an inherited genetic problem.)

Eventually I came down with severe stomach cramps. I went to a doctor who sent me to the M. Hospital, where I had received an intravenous polygram of my kidneys and gall bladder, X-rays and a complete G.I. series. The kidneys, stomach and gall bladder were normal, but there were pus cells in the urine. They called in a urologist who gave me a cystoscopic examination. He found two small stones in my left kidney and bacillus coli infection in my prostate gland. I was discharged from the hospital and was told to take four antibiotics per day while I waited for the results of the urine culture that had been sent to Hartford.

The results confirmed what the urologist had suspected; I had tuberculosis in my left kidney. I was given medications that I had to take for two years to kill the full cycle of the T.B. germs. My wife gave me 2 cc's injections of streptomycin twice a week for two years, and I took ten tablets of para-amino salicyclic acid three times per day and another white tablet, the name of which I have forgotten, three times per day—which made thirty-three in all.

From then on all further culture tests came back negative, which meant that I was completely free of T.B.

In the meantime, my arthritis was still raising havoc with my spine, which was gradually growing less flexible. I went to see a doctor in New Haven who was recommended to me by a friend I worked with.

His name was Dr. B., a man in his late sixties with iron-gray hair and bushy eyebrows who, I learned later, hated blacks and women, especially if they were nurses. He gave me a complete examination and then, with great confidence, told me he could cure my arthritis because of a new medication called Aristicort that showed great promise.

He went so far as to say that Aristicort would not only dissolve the "chalk" around my spine, but it would also dissolve the stones in my kidney. I was elated by this good news and Stephanie and I left his office floating on cloud nine. In addition to Aristicort, Dr. B. had also prescribed Nicotinic Acid and gave me a B-12 injection at every visit.

I must admit that over the following months I was not only free of arthritic pains, but my movements in general became much swifter and I felt a lot more limber. My confidence in this racist, Dr. B., went up considerably, even though I did not like him as a person very much.

About a year later, with my activity and endurance having increased to my normal pre-arthritis days, to my chagrin I began experiencing severe muscle spasms in my back. I phoned Dr. B. and was taken aback by his joyful reaction. He was actually very delighted that my back was acting up. He said this meant that Aristicort was working, the "chalk" around my spine was dissolving giving my spine greater motion, and the dormant muscles were merely reacting to these new movements. Once the muscles adjusted to the new movements the spasms would vanish, and he prescribed Darvon to help me endure the terrible pain.

Some six months later, the incredibly painful spasms still continued and Dr. B. told me they would continue till my spine was completely free of "chalk." He prescribed Indocin, one capsule three times per day for pain, and Empirin Compound, two tablets every two or three hours.

Later, when I pointed out to him that Empirin had a warning label that said it could cause possible kidney damage, Dr. B. pooh-poohed the warning as so much more medical nonsense. His cavalier-like attitude toward the warnings cause me to have second thoughts about him, so I decided to reduce the Empirin dosage on my own.

The two student nurses went on scribbling in their notebooks. I continued.

A couple of months later, I came down with a stubborn case of diarrhea with watery stools that were very dark in color. I felt lethargic, but continued working, thinking it was all merely a mild case of the flu.

On Saturday, while I was at home, I found blood in my stools. I phoned Dr. B., who told me that without other symptoms he did not think it significant. He suggested I take mineral oil for a few days to lubricate the bowels. He believed the bleeding may have been due to a scratch from a fish bone or some other sharp food substance. (I had not eaten fish in over a month.)

I convinced myself that there was nothing to worry about, yet I did not feel well. There was a strange tenseness and restlessness that I had never felt before. I lay down for a short nap, and when I got up I felt groggy. I put on my winter jacket and went out to the cold and windy backyard for a walk, then came back into the house feeling nauseous. I sat down on the living room couch, and it got worse.

The nausea became even more intense. I stood up, and as a sudden dizzyness came over me, I reached out my hand for support, but I don't think I found it because I suddenly lost consciousness. Stephanie, who had been watching, told me later that I had fallen flat on my back with a loud bang that shook the whole house.

When I came to, it was like waking from a deep sleep. I was able to hear Stephanie, as if in a dream, frantically trying to phone for an ambulance. The M. Hospital told her they had no ambulances and that she would have to get her own. She then phoned Dr. O'D., a local doctor, who told her to let me lie on the floor for at least ten minutes before letting me get up. After I got up, I immediately went to the bathroom where I passed more black stools.

In a few minutes, Dr. O'D. arrived at our home. He took my blood pressure and told me not to move from the couch I lay on, then phoned the M. Hospital for me to be admitted immediately. That was when I first learned that black stools meant that bleeding was occurring in the stomach.

After seven days in the hospital, restricted from Aristicort, I was back on my feet and working again.

About a month later the muscle spasms became unbearably painful. They had become more frequent, of longer duration, and came during the day and night. They were causing me loss of sleep and loss of energy, and they were wearing me out at work.

The agony was unbelievable. In the full grip of a spasm I felt as though I were being run over by a tractor-trailer fully loaded. The only way I could get some blessed relief was by laying on a heating pad which I could only do when I was at home.

I phoned Dr. B. about my desperate situation and he told me to take two Indocin capsules at one time when necessary for pain, in addition to the Empirin tablets.

A couple of months later I told Dr. B. that my elbows, knees and ankles were growing stiff. He said it was due to the same disease and the Aristicort that I was still taking would help the other joints.

Despite the medication, my joints were just getting worse and I found it impossible to continue working and to carry out my duties as Union Shop Steward. Therefore, I resigned my stewardship and on the following day I took a leave of absence from work.

I went to see Dr. O'D. about my weight loss and completely run-down condition. He suspected that I had either a recurrence of TB or possibly some hidden cancer, and I was sent to M. Hospital.

At the hospital I was placed in isolation and given X-rays and other tests. Stephanie and other visitors had to put on white gowns and masks over their mouths and noses. After ten days, with all tests proving negative, I was finally discharged.

Since nothing had been done for my underweight and run-down condition and my back spasms, I went to a local orthopedic surgeon, who after several X-rays and a half dozen visits prescribed a corset for me to wear.

After passing the company doctor's physical examination and signing a waiver for my back, I returned to work. The corset I was wearing made my work days more comfortable and almost spasm free.

But a few weeks later I again came down with stomach bleeding, which Dr. O'D. managed to control with antacids and a special diet. I did not have to lose any more time from work.

My right knee, which had been swollen for a long time, began to grow painful at work. My left hip was also getting painful and I began using a cane to help me walk.

Soon after that I was fired for writing an article for a New Haven newsletter that criticized union-company collusion.

Because Stephanie was still working, we managed to survive. But, in the meantime, my condition continued to worsen, and I discontinued wearing the constricting corset.

Stephanie and I headed back to Dr. B.'s office. I had been off Aristicort for over three months because of the stomach bleeding I had had. I was looking forward to being put back on Aristicort so that I could get some relief from my pain and stiffness. But when we got there we found his door closed. A woman from across the hall told us that Dr. B. had died. I was stunned, not so much that he had died, but mostly because he had died without letting me know about it. I felt like a drug addict who desperately needed a "fix" and was suddenly cut off from his source and knew not where else to turn.

The woman gave us the name and address of a Dr. H., also in New Haven.

After making an appointment, Stephanie and I had gone to his office and he gave me a complete physical examination. Then, back at his desk, he told us that mine was a complicated case. The kidney stones could be caused by a rheumatoid factor he said. The stomach bleeding required that I stay away from certain medications, especially Aristicort, and a combination of other things. Until all these things were thoroughly looked into, he could not come up with a definite treatment. Also he wanted to look at all my X-rays taken at M. Hospital. He wanted me to bring them to him on my next visit to his office. In the meantime he gave me thirty tablets of Ascriptin to hold me over till then.

While Stephanie worked, on my next visit, I drove myself to Dr. H.'s office only to learn that he could not come up with anything in terms of treatment. "That's the state of the art," he said. Then he added that his choice of drugs for me were very limited, and prescribed sixteen tablets of Ascriptin per day (which were of little help), plus some simple exercises to help me walk straighter. I left his office very disappointed, yet I sensed that he knew what he was doing.

Unlike Dr. B., Dr. H. did not promise any magic "cure." Although Dr. H. had not helped me much, at least he had done me no harm, so far. Dr. B., on the other hand, not only had worsened my arthritis, he had also caused me to be hospitalized for stomach bleeding. Yet, despite my misgivings, I foolishly continued going back to him because I was too desperate to think rationally. I was grasping for help, any kind of help, and therefore I strongly wanted to believe in him.

Sometime later a strange thing occurred. I had been lying on my back on the living room carpet reading a newspaper for half an hour, as I usually did to keep my spine from curling. When I got up, I was surprised at how easily I did it and at how straight and free of pain I was when I walked. It was unbelievable, as if I had been touched by a magic wand that washed away all my arthritis. I was so elated that I went outside in the back yard and walked around without effort or pain, and for the first time in a long time I was able to enjoy the rustic surroundings. Before this, the painful struggle to propel myself from one point to another was so great that the song birds and the various colors of the surrounding vegetation receded into oblivion as far as I was concerned. Now I enjoyed the environment, life was again beautiful and inspiring. Raw energy surged through me and intoxicated me with exhilarating enthusiasm. It was indeed a miracle!

But unfortunately, the next day the miracle ended.

On my next visit to Dr. H.'s office he sent me to a medical laboratory for a number of blood tests, all of which came back negative except one for severe anemia. He prescribed Vitron-C for me.

A few days later I received a phone call from Dr. H. He told me he still did not know how to treat me. There were many questions that had to be answered. The most pressing one was: Exactly what was causing my anemia? He suggested I go to the veterans hospital for complete tests. I balked at the idea of being hospitalized. He said we would talk about it some other time. In the meantime, he wanted to talk to the urologist who did the cystoscopic examination of my kidneys at M. Hospital about the slight changes in my recent kidney X-rays.

When my next blood test results came in, Dr. H. told me there was no improvement in my anemia, and that my sedimentation rate of over a hundred was very high, indicating some kind of infectious activity. In the latest kidney X-rays, a small pocket near the top of my left kidney showed some changes. It might be TB, but because it was not connected to a urine outlet, no germs had been detected in my urine. He again suggested I go to a veterans hospital to get these things investigated to confirm it one way or another. Since I was out of work this would be the cheapest way to do this, and I would be in the hospital for only three weeks.

This time I consented.

When a bed was available Stephanie drove me to a large Veterans Administration hospital. We went to the Admittance Office, where a woman at the desk asked me a number of questions. Then I handed her my Army Discharge papers to verify that I was a veteran who had served during wartime. When all the paperwork had been completed, she sent us to Building #2 on the fourth floor, where I was installed in a room with two beds, and a nurse took my vital signs.

Later a young intern came in and took my medical history. After changing into pajamas I went to the examining room where the intern gave me a complete physical examination.

After supper I went out to the hall and phoned Stephanie. When I got back to my room another doctor had come in. He listened to my heart, then told me that the next day I would get bone marrow drawn from my hip bone.

In the evening, besides my other medication, I received two sleeping pills. Although I was very sleepy I found it impossible to fall asleep because my hips were aching. I was not accustomed to the bed, and there was a strange restlessness in my legs. I got up frequently to walk through the silent hallways. It was not till 3:30 A.M. that I finally fell asleep.

I was up at 7 A.M. After breakfast I was sent to the first floor, where I had two vials of blood drawn, then I went back to my room where I slept for about an hour.

After dinner the doctor came in with a young woman assistant. I was instructed to lie on the bed on my left side, then with Bethedine and alcohol the doctor swabbed a wide area of my right hip and injected a novocaine supply into my hip. After that he was handed a syringe with a long needle attached to it. He pushed the needle through my skin and into the hip bone, where he had to exert great pressure to gradually work it deeper and deeper into the hard bone. I was experiencing not only the pressure pains but also the fear that the needle would break inside the bone.

The needle continued moving down into my bone for what seemed like an inordinately long time. Finally, when I felt a sharp jerking pain, I relaxed a little, thinking the needle had broken through, but the doctor told me he still had another quarter of an inch to go yet. At last it broke through the bone into the marrow cavity from which the doctor drew out a sample. I finally relaxed, and the young nurse pricked my finger with a small needle and put some drops of blood on a couple of glass slides.

The doctor put a bandaid on my hip and told me it had gone a little harder than usual because my bones were more dense because of arthritis. He added that one needle had bent on the way in, but it all went well.

For weeks I was sent to Hematology for more blood tests and X-rays, and many doctors and student doctors kept coming into my room to examine me and to ask me the same old tired questions, over and over again. And when it was discovered that I had an enlarged spleen, even more doctors from all over came just to feel my spleen. But, because it would help the medical profession, I cheerfully allowed it all to go on. At first they wanted to remove the spleen, but when they found that it was not causing me any harm, they decided not to.

The tests continued, and so did the urine collections, dental X-rays, brain X-rays, and, of course, the blood tests.

The doctor came in with the results of the bone marrow test, and he told me my bone marrow was producing red blood cells more efficiently than average. But not fast enough to provide for my special needs. Despite all the tests, they still did not know exactly where my red blood cells were being lost. The spleen was one possibility, TB in my kidney was another. They had found some abnormalities in the preliminary urine tests, and further study was still necessary. The doctor stuck a plastic tube into my nose, down to my stomach, and drew out some fluids for a TB culture. Then I had more blood drawn from my arm. If they had put an end to my daily blood tests, perhaps my anemia would not be so serious, I thought after he had left.

Later the nurse told me to report to Radio Isotopes immediately. As I walked toward the smaller building behind the two large buildings, I was followed by a dark shadow of trepidation that graduated to outright anguish as I wondered whether they had found a fatal cancer in me, which they would try to treat with radioactivity.

When I got there I learned to my relief that they were merely going to check my red blood cells for longevity. Normal cells usually live about thirty days.

The technician drew a vial of blood from my arm, then told me to return at a specific time.

When I returned to my room the nurse told me to report to the heart station for an electro-cardiogram. From there I went back to Radio Isotopes. There a doctor reinjected my blood into my vein. The blood was now radioactive. He told me to return again at a specific time.

When I returned to Radio Isotopes a technician withdrew

two vials of blood, and that was the end of that test.

The doctors still had not come up with any definitive answer to my problems. I was still going to Physical Therapy to soak in the Hubbard tub and exercise my arms in the Therapy Room with overhead pulleys, and making frequent trips to the Canteen to buy giant chocolate bars and other snacks, besides my regular meals, to satiate my voracious appetite.

I had been getting iron supplements and the doctor told me my blood count had gone up a little, which was a good sign.

My blood pressure had been 120/70 for many years and it still was at that level despite all the tests which brought me tension and anguish. At breakfast I was now getting three eggs and two slices of bacon to try to cut down some of my fierce hunger.

The tests continued ad nauseam and the next report was that they were still trying to determine whether to keep giving me iron pills or whether to give me iron injections. Also, my kidneys indicated some kind of infectious activity, but even if it were TB, it still would not explain the whole anemia problem. My case was very complicated, they said.

I had a prostate biopsy in which a piece of the prostate gland was sniped off.

When I got back to my room I had to make frequent trips to the bathroom to empty my bowels of red blood. I told the nurse, who merely cancelled my Physical Therapy appointment. The bleeding continued and I again told the nurse. She looked into the toilet bowl and said it looked like a lot of blood but was actually only a few teaspoonfuls. I was not reassured.

I went to bed at 11 P.M., but during the night I was up at least eight times dumping blood into the toilet bowl.

At 7 A.M., on my way back from the bathroom, I suddenly

felt dizzy and everything around me began to grow dim, and the nerve endings in my legs screamed with a silent vibrational sensation.

No one was around me and I slowly made my way to the nearest chair, which was in the nurses' station, where I sat back with my eyes closed against the fading of my vision and the marked weakness.

A nurse brought me back to my room in a wheelchair, helped me into bed and told me not to leave it for any reason.

I had breakfast in bed, afterwhich the doctor came in to check my pulse and looked under my eye lids.

Later I had an I.V. put into a vein in my arm and a unit of whole blood and a bottle of saline solution slowly flowed into my bloodstream. The doctor told me I would receive two units of blood to replace what I had lost. He also cancelled my weekend pass, which disappointed me.

Sometime later, I had five vials of blood drawn instead of the two or three vials they had usually drawn.

Still later I had two vials of blood drawn at Radio Isotopes. Back in my room the doctor took a couple of saliva samples onto three glass slides. Then three doctors came to examine me, being particularly interested in the completely diminished hair on my arms and legs.

A couple of days later I had an Intravenous Polygram (IVP) done on my kidneys. As usual a couple of the X-rays had to be done over again because they did not develop clearly.

I was scheduled for another IVP. This time the iodine would be slowly "dripped" into my kidneys. After going through all the preliminaries, which included Castor Oil, two enemas and a missed breakfast, the nurse told me the IVP was cancelled.

The IVP was rescheduled, I received a large dose of Castor Oil and again I was told the IVP was cancelled. Later they apologetically told me, after I had eaten supper, that it was not the IVP, but rather the liver isotopes X-rays that had been cancelled.

"Were you angry?" the two students asked me, and I affirmed that I was. I was anxious to get these tests over with by giving my complete cooperation, but all I had been getting from them was chaos and confusion. Three shifts of nurses and doctors, from various departments, with no or bad communications among each other, were probably the biggest factor in most of the confusion.

At last I was actually on the table in X-ray. The doctor had mixed the dye in a pint of saline solution, then he stuck the needle in an arm vein, and in about 15 or 20 minutes of slow dripping the bottle was empty. The X-ray technician took some exposures, then a series of laminations. After they were developed the doctor told me the kidney stones in my left kidney were smaller than a dime. To me that seemed quite large since only a month earlier they had been insignificant.

A few days later I was back in the X-ray Department. This time I came in a wheelchair feeling stiff as a plank of oak because I had had no medication for my arthritis. The grueling upper G.I. series consisted of my drinking five large cups of berium, while being fluoroscoped, gagging on the fifth cup. After that I was X-rayed in another room where a couple of exposures had to be done over again.

After breakfast the doctor told me that my kidney X-rays revealed only the kidney stones but no infectious activity. My red blood count of 26 remained stable but the iron injections should bring it up. He also added that I had no ulcer, and the kidney stones were situated in a position where they could not be removed. They decided that the liver biopsy they had been planning was no longer necessary. He explained that I lost blood from taking aspirins, from the kidney stone irritations and from the inflammation in my knees. Also, the kidney stones were in both kidneys, although in the right kidney the stones were very tiny. To keep them from growing any larger, they suggested that I drink a lot of water every day.

A few days later the nurse told me to report to the fifth floor conference room. All my doctors, including my outside doctor, H., were there. Some of my X-rays were stuck up on the light panels, and I stood there before them like an inmate facing a Parole Board for the crime of getting arthritis, and I answered their questions.

In any event, on Friday the doctor told me the delightful news that I was discharged. Anxious as I was to get the hell out of there I quickly dressed into my street clothes. After a lot of mix-ups and red tape, I was finally driving homeward feeling free as an uncaged wild animal. Yet, because I still had the arthritis, I sensed an ominous cloud following me and, when my mind shifted back to the hospital, an uncertain anger and dismay seized me. I just could not believe that I had been hospitalized for three months when Dr. H. had told me it would be only three weeks! I had gone through all those horrendouus tests and not a damn thing more had been learned than before I had gone to the hospital. Three lousy months of pain and anguish and all for nothing, absolutely nothing! And HINDSIGHT told me, in no uncertain terms, that I was a stupid fool for allowing all that to happen to me.

All this I had narrated to the two student nurses and they occasionally interrupted me to ask questions. They told me that I was very helpful, their report on arthritis would weigh heavily on the grades they get at the University of Bridgeport, and they asked me if I would allow them to come back for more information. I replied that they could and they left with their notes and happy smiles on their faces.

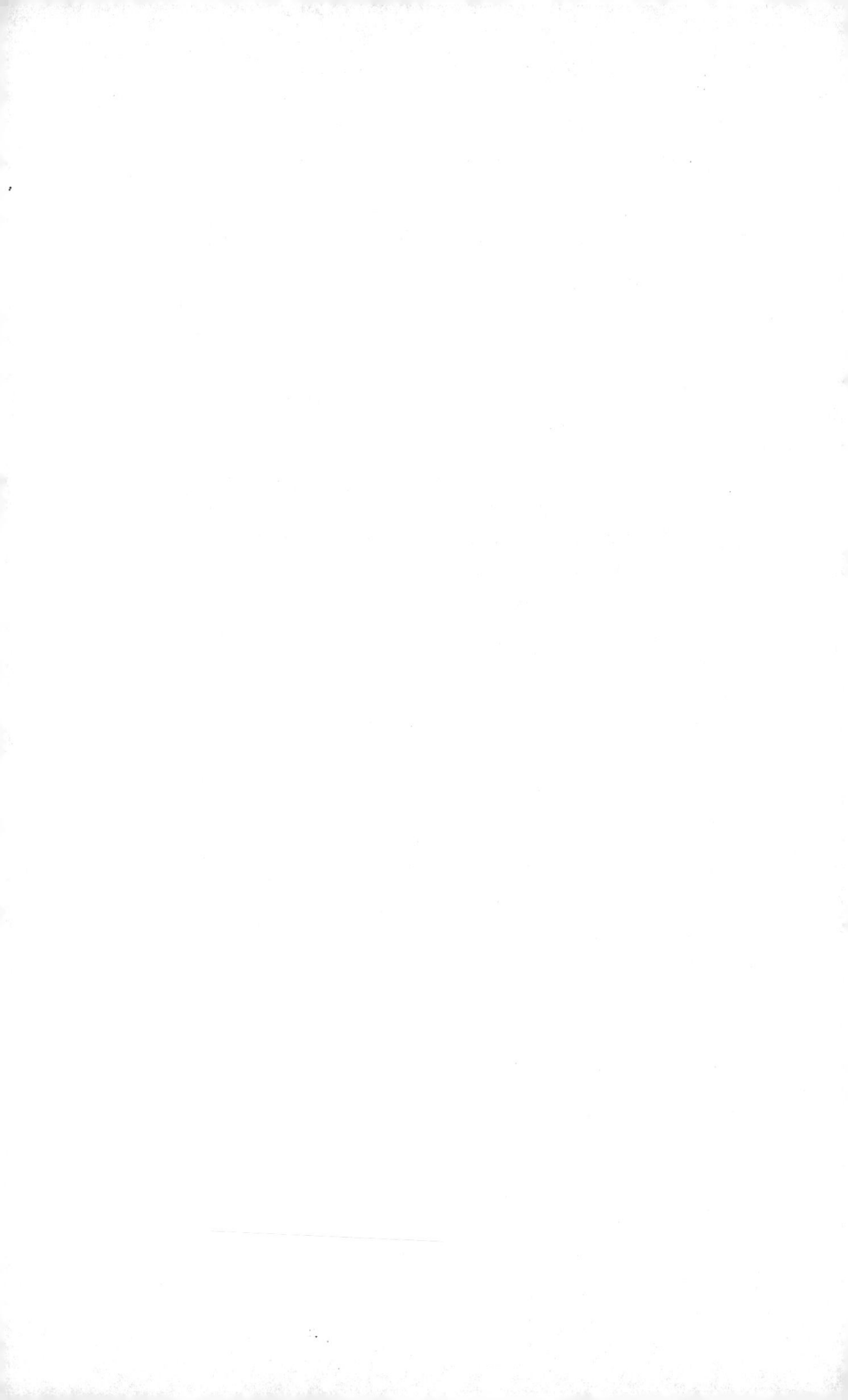

Chapter 4

Two weeks later, the two student nurses returned to my house. They wanted to know how the arthritis had effected me psychologically, and a little more of my background.

I explained to them that psychologically the arthritis did not disturb me very much in the earlier years of my disease. I ignored the pain, which I had managed to control by consuming large amounts of aspirin, and by constantly being active in such things as jogging a few laps around my back yard, participating in municipal and state politics and in labor union organizing, and being elected Shop Steward where I worked. Somehow in back of my mind I always believed that I would some day overcome the disease, simply through sheer orneriness and an undying optimism.

Even when the arthritis invaded my hip joints, I still kept going, paying only cursory attention to the tightness in my hips. At work, when I was on union business, I often had to climb three flights of stairs some four or five times a day to cover all the workers I represented, and I always skipped easily up the stairs in a running jog. However, when the stiffness came to my hips I found myself getting winded, so I cut down on my pipe smoking which I had been doing constantly for ten years. But over the months I began using the hand railings to help pull myself up what felt like Mount

Everest. The hip joints slowed me down considerably and I sometimes worried about it but, as long as I was still performing my duties, I did not allow it to depress me.

Then I described to the two student nurses how all through my horrendous hospital tests and hip surgery I had continued to maintain my optimism—surviving the hospital made surviving my arthritis child's play.

All during the process of the disease I had asked myself why this had happened to me. Many times I had gone back over my life, reminiscing, pondering, speculating and searching for some clue that would unlock this mystery.

Among the outstanding traumas and incidents in my life which I had suspected as contributors to my present woes were:

When I was nine years old during the height of the 1930's Depression, I came down with what was diagnosed as pneumonia. I was hospitalized as a charity case and the X-rays discovered that I had Empyema. During my year in the hospital I hovered between life and death and was frequently X-rayed, and operated on three times. I was nothing but skin and bones and, before each operation, the parish priest would come to visit me with his candles, cotton and oils to give me the last rites. I confessed to him each time that I had stolen some playing marbles from a neighborhood kid, which was the only sin I could think of in those days. Of course, I believed him when he told me I would go to heaven, but at age nine, I just was not interested in going to heaven so soon. Every weekend and on Wednesdays, my parents would come to the children's ward to visit me. I was bedridden and could not even be near them to talk to and to touch them. The ward was sectioned off by panels of metal and glass with four patients to each cubicle. On visiting days the entrance to each cubicle was chained off so that my parents had to lean on their elbows on the heavy chain and shout to communicate with me, and I, with a heavy heart, watched the river of tears running down my father's anguished face as he sobbed uncontrollably. My mother was a more practical person who had a no-nonsense approach to hard living, yet she too occasionally dabbed her handkerchief over her tearful eyes. I felt terrible that I was causing them so much pain and I tried to cheer them up as much as I could. But being helplessly imprisoned in a sick body, I knew that the only way I would be able to alleviate their pain was either to get better or to die. But dying was just not on my agenda, so my only other alternative was that I would have to get better, which had been my full intention all along.

Each of the three times I had gone to surgery the doctors opened a new site to put in a drainage tube to drain pus from my left back chest cavity in the area between the rib cage and the lungs. (They had no antibiotics in those days.)

Gradually over the months the infection slowed down to a trickle, and the drainage tube, which ran down into a gallon jug hanging low on the side of my bed, was removed and a short catheter was inserted in its place and covered over with bandages and tape. This had freed me from my bed, allowing me to get out of bed into a wheelchair and to learn how to walk again. Then I was discharged from the hospital.

We lived in a cold-water flat on the second floor in the slum area of East Side Bridgeport. Though I was able to walk I was still in no condition to climb the stairs on my own. I depended on my parents to carry me on their backs up the creaky wood stairs. Since I was vastly underweight it was not too difficult for each of them to do it. Also, I was too weak to go with my brother Joe to play with the neighborhood boys, so I would sit on the front porch stairs with our family dog, Jackie, on my lap, stroking its shaggy fur and waiting for my father to come home from the boiler works where he was finally employed again after a long shut-down. When I would see him some two blocks away, Jackie and I would walk toward him and meet him a block away. He would smile happily and ask me what I had achieved that day and we would talk as we walked. Jackie's tail wagged wildly, and when we reached our house, my father happily carried me up the stairs on his sturdy back. His face and clothes were blackened with soot, and he would remove his shirt and wash himself with a washcloth from a large pan of hot water my mother had prepared on the kitchen stove.

When I finally managed to climb the stairs on my own it was a happy day for all of us. A doctor told my parents that my weight was not going up and he suggested that I get some meat at least twice a week so that I could catch up with the rest of my brothers and sisters. My father earned $18.00 per week and I felt guilty when I had meat for supper while everyone else in the family was eating various Slovak meals without meat. When I finally regained my weight I went back on the same high-starch diet that the rest of the family was eating. Eventually the short drainage tube in my back was removed, the incision healed and I was fully recovered and bounding with unlimited energy.

The two student nurses wanted to know whether the Empyema had ever returned and how I got along after that.

I told them that it never returned again and that all through my teenage years my brother Joe and I participated in all the rough-and-tumble activities in the neighborhood. My muscles grew hard and I felt light as a ping-pong ball and could not resist leap-frogging over fire hydrants and stop signs. Even the highest stop sign did not deter me. As long as I was able to reach the top of the sign with my hands, I would simply run up to it and grab it while I sprang up like a cat and, with the support of my hands, would smoothly glide over it.

Also during my early teen years, my brother Joe and I each

built a shoeshine box and went downtown to shine shoes for nickles and dimes. We also had newspaper routes and we worked as pin-setters in a bowling alley.

When I turned sixteen I went to the State Trade School during the day, and on the evenings and weekends I worked at the bowling alleys. It was there, after long hours of constant bending, that I experienced my first backaches. But the backaches were only due to exertion and soon vanished when we got home. Yet, when I looked back, I wondered whether these exertions may have been planting the seeds for my spinal arthritis.

Also, in 1943, at age eighteen, I was drafted into the Army. I was not too thrilled with the Infantry so I took some extra physical tests and managed to get into the Army Air Corps for pilot training. Instead I ended up as a radio operator on B-29's. Climbing into a bomber that had been sitting in the hot sun was like getting into a hot oven. Under these high temperatures each crew member did his respective preflight inspection, and when that was completed we would take off and soon be at 35,000 feet in below-zero temperatures. Our aircraft was pressurized and warm, but my radio equipment was right next to the door of the forward bomb bay, which was not pressurized and was quite chilly. Although it had no physical effect on me at that time, I had read that rapid temperature changes were often linked to arthritis.

Also, I was exposed to radiation from the first atomic bomb explosion in White Sands, New Mexico, which was about fifteen miles from our air base in Alamagordo. We were sleeping in our barracks when the early morning explosion shook the ground like a small earthquake. Later, because of our curiosity, we flew low over the greenish-blue crater, not knowing a thing about the dangers of radiation. I believe this experience also had contributed to my present woes.

After the war ended, even though I was a tool-and-die maker, I discovered that jobs were hard to find. I worked for a while in a buckle factory, which did not satisfy me. I quit and joined the Merchant Marines, and sailed as an ordinary seaman on an old liberty ship named Zebulan B. Vance. On one trip coming back from Bremerhaven, Germany, we sailed along the North Sea route. The seas were rough and the winds icy. Yet I did my four hours on and eight hours off standing watch on the icy deck of the ship's bow completely undaunted. Here again, it had no physical effect on me at that time, but the prolonged exposure to the extreme cold temperatures may have been still another factor paving the way to my current problems.

After leaving the Merchant Marines I went into the retail frozen-food business. I took out a bank loan and bought a truck with a refrigerator body. Selling frozen foods from house to house required climbing in and out of the refrigerator at every stop. During the winter months I always wore heavy clothing, but during the hot summer months I wore a short-sleeve shirt. Although I had a jacket to put on every time I entered the refrigerator, I found it to be too much of a nuisance, so most of the time I would not wear it. Looking back at this alternating warmth and chill, I wondered how much damage I might have incurred to my entire system that subsequently led to my arthritis.

When the frozen-food business failed due to my lack of business knowledge and equipment failures, I had the refrigerator taken off and a straight rack body put on in its place. With the new truck body I joined the Teamsters Union and began hauling freight. This required loading my own truck at factory shipping platforms, driving to the freight's destination, then unloading the freight. It was strenuous work, but it was nothing I could not handle.

After a year and many truck breakdowns, I procured a job

with the National Transportation Company driving tractor-trailers. Here again, besides the long hours of driving, I often had to load and unload the trailer. It was heavy work and, although I was 5'9" and weighed 158 pounds, I was lifting and handling heavy freight that large musclebound men were struggling with, and I had more stamina. Most of my work days were as long as twelve hours. But after three and a half years, I began feeling backaches at night, so I quit to go back to my trade in a factory.

All these incidents taken together, I believed, could very well have triggered off the Ankylosing Spondylitis, I told the two student nurses. They thanked me for this new information, then they left.

A couple of months later I came down with another episode of stomach bleeding which was not too serious. The doctor in the Emergency Room suggested I take Tylenol instead of aspirin. I did so and within a week the bleeding stopped.

Stephanie stayed home from work to go with me to my next Arthritis Clinic appointment. A woman doctor listened to my heart, then drew four vials of blood to test my kidney functions. Then she called in Dr. C., who came in with two young doctors. I walked around the room so the two young interns could try to diagnose me. After a few bad guesses they came up with Ankylosing Spondylitis. C. said that while steroid injections in my right knee would help it, they could also damage it over prolonged periods, and it was best not to resort to them unless absolutely necessary.

A few weeks later at the Arthritis Clinic my blood pressure was 185/107 and I was definitely concerned about it. After a short wait, it was taken again and was 155/98, which was still high. But the fact that it had come down a little indicated that it was just apprehension, the doctor said. I did not feel apprehensive when I had come in, so I felt that these sudden rises in my blood pressure were due to a new and still mysterious development. My arthritis was fairly stable and, after the routine examination, I left.

About six months later, Dr. R. invited me to come to the hospital and speak before an audience of nurses. Dr. R. met me in the lobby and we took the elevator to the ninth floor and went into the auditorium where I was introduced to the "scrub" nurse who was responsible for keeping the operating room germ-free. A large number of nurses then came in, and Dr. R. got up to the podium and spoke about the history of the hip operation. After that he showed some slides of an elderly man, before and after his hip surgery. He also showed one slide of me on a stretcher in the operating room just before surgery. Then he introduced me to the audience and I spoke about my problems before surgery and the excellent results after. This was followed by an informal demonstration of how the powdered glue was mixed with a catalyst in a plastic bowl and stirred until it became doughy and generated some heat. We also handled and examined the prosthesis and the tapered rasp-boring tool and other instruments. Then we watched a film of an actual hip replacement operation. It was quite a gruesome sight. After that the meeting ended.

In a February snow storm in 1974, I was trying to start a stubborn snow blower and inadvertently twisted my left hip and felt a dull clumping sound. The next day I could not straighten my leg at the hip, and it was painful to walk on. I phoned Dr. R. and described to him what had happened. He said I might have dislocated it, but that it had gone back in place because I was able to move it in all directions.

Stephanie drove me to the hospital where I had my hips X-rayed per Dr. R.'s orders. When the films were ready Dr. R. checked them against those that I had taken just two weeks earlier and said there was no change. There was a large hematoma on the thigh near the injured hip. He said it was consistent with what had happened. He examined my leg motions and checked the pulse in my left foot, which he said was good and strong. He believed I might have torn a muscle when I twisted the ball joint out, and there was about a pint of blood that had collected in the upper thigh which was the hematoma. He said it would disperse and gradually disappear.

In the meantime I was leading a fairly active and busy life, writing a labor column for *Modern Times*, teaching American labor history for the Park City Alternative at the University of Bridgeport, and participating in anti-war rallies and demonstrations along with Stephanie.

In the summer of 1975 I found that my urine had become cloudy with a light-colored substance. After a week of waiting I phoned the V.A. Emergency Room, and was told to come right down.

When I got there they wanted a sterile urine sample, which I gave them. Then a nurse told me to check in so that I could get my chart. After a long hassle, I finally got my chart and brought it to the the Emergency Room. After a long wait, I was told to take the chart to someone else at the end of the hall. There, a woman took it and asked me to sit in a chair, then she left. When she got back, she asked me to sit in the waiting room. After another long wait, a nurse called me into one of the empty rooms, asked me about my problem, then checked my vital signs. My blood pressure was 190/100. This time I realized what I had suspected, that my blood pressure was not up due to stress. In the past stress never effected my blood pressure very much. I had an uneasy feeling that this was something more drastic then simple hypertension. What was happening to me was something sinister and ominous, and it had something to do with my recent tiredness and the cloudy urine.

Anyway, she wrote an order for blood tests and X-rays.

After I had three vials of blood drawn, I went to the X-ray Department, where I waited, only to be told that they were jammed up with people; so I went to the other building, where I again waited a very long time because one of their X-ray machines was not working properly.

In the meantime, I sat there completely exhausted and demoralized, wondering whether or not they would find something fatal in me, which kept me in a constant state of worry. Finally, I got on the X-ray table and had my hips X-rayed. But when the film was developed, it came out too dark, so I had to get it done over again, adding disgust to my other feelings.

I carried the X-ray films back to Building #1, where I gave them to a nurse who told me to sit in the waiting room. After another long wait, I was called into the Examining Room. The doctor phoned the lab and was told there was blood in my urine, but not a lot. He explained that it took only a little blood to produce cloudy urine. He then phoned a urologist who made an appointment with me, and I finally left.

Each time I went to the V.A. Clinic, I saw an increased evidence that the reduced staff was unable to cope with the heavy patient load, and conditions for everyone continued to deteriorate. I once went to the clinic to get my urine analyzed, but this simple procedure was accomplished only after five tension and anguish-filled hours.

A week later I went to the Urology Clinic. After I was called in, the doctor asked me how long I had had blood in the urine. I told him that I had it, on rare occasions, for about fifteen years. Usually it had a pink or reddish tinge to it and it lasted only about a couple of hours, but this was the first time I had cloudy urine that continued for about two weeks. He suggested that I get admitted for a couple of days for an I.V.P. and a cystoscopic examination of my bladder.

A few days later I was admitted to the hospital. My blood

pressure was 200/110, and the nurse said it was nothing but tension. "Lots of people have high blood pressure when they first get admitted," she added. My blood pressure had always been 120/70, even on all my prior hospital admittances, but I did not want to argue with her.

In the evening I received a bottle of Evac-Q-Mag to drink. Later I received two Evac-Q tablets. And still later a suppository. During the night I had several bowel movements and in the morning, at 6 A.M., I received another suppository.

At 8 A.M. I was in X-ray, where three preliminary exposures were made. The doctor came in, told me the X-rays were not clear because my bowels were not completely empty, and I was sent back upstairs. An hour later I was called down again. After a long wait, I finally got on the table and had one exposure made. Then, off the table, standing up, I had two views of my chest done. Then back to the waiting room I went, only to be told that my bowels were still not clear. I was exasperated by all this stupid jostling and unnecessary exposure to X-rays, and I wondered why they had given me Evac-Q-Mag, which did not work on me, instead of the traditional Castor Oil and enemas that always did work on me.

In the evening, I went through the same Evac-Q-Mag procedure, and in the morning I was back in X-ray only to be told that an emergency case had come in. I was sent back upstairs to keep fasting and to wait for their call.

About an hour later, I was back on the table in X-ray where two exposures were made which finally turned out to be all right. A gray-haired doctor with an East-European accent placed a needle into a vein in my arm, then injected the iodine dye. There was a cool feeling as the dye went into my vein, followed by a warm glow that came over my whole body. The doctor asked me if I was all right. I said I was. Four exposures were made at five-minute intervals. Then exposures were taken of my left side, then of my right side. After that I was told to empty out my bladder and more exposures were taken.

I went back to my ward and quenched my thirst. In the afternoon I was sent to a room which had a table surrounded by a variety of strange machinery for my cystoscopic examination. Feeling apprehensive, I lay back on the table with a male attendant's help, and my legs were placed wide part in stirrups. My pubic areas were swabbed with Bethadine and my legs and belly were covered with gray-green sterile cloths. Then he injected Lydicaine into my penis passageway (urethra) to make it numb.

Then the urologist came in wearing the green operating room garb which his attendant also wore. The doctor slowly inserted a long thin instrument with a light on the end into my urethra. Then, through the other end, he looked into the eye-piece and moved the instrument through various angles. At this point another doctor came in and also looked into the eye piece. In the meantime, from a bottle hanging on a pole, saline solution was draining into my bladder to expand it. They took turns examining my bladder and the passageway (ureter) to my kidneys, which was quite an uncomfortable pulling sensation along with the discomfort of the saline-filled bladder. I was very happy when it was finally all over.

The doctor told me there were no changes in the I.V.P., the bladder looked alright, and that I could go home—which made me even happier.

I hurried to the bathroom to empty out my bladder but, to my dismay, I passed only a tiny bit, and was shut off by a strange gurgling sound followed by two drops of blood. Yet this goshawful urge to urinate still remained with me.

I told the nurse about my inability to urinate. She called the doctor, who told me that the reason was because they had completely drained the bladder and he suggested that I drink a lot of water. Why didn't the idiot tell me that in the first place? I said to myself. Anyway, he also added that I had a slight infection in my urinary tract and prescribed Macradantin for it, and added that if I passed urine, then I could go home.

After drinking plenty of water, I passed a lot of urine and was discharged.

A few weeks later Stephanie went with me to the hypertension clinic. There were many patients ahead of me. After a long wait, a nurse called me into one of the rooms and took my blood pressure, which was 200/110. She gave me a list of tests I had to get: blood test, urine sample, chest X-rays and an E.K.G.

After getting all the tests done, I returned with Stephanie and waited endlessly till the doctor came in. He had my chart and asked me a number of questions. Then he gave me a complete physical examination, including my eyes, which he dilated with eye drops. He said that, although my blood pressure was up, there were no complications. He explained the mild treatment he would give me for fifteen days. If the blood pressure came down I might not need further treatment, or I might need two or three fifteen-day treatments. He prescribed Lasix, two mg. daily, with orange juice or any other fruit juices with high potassium because Lasix washed potassium out of the body.

After that, I had to get admitted at the downstairs office, then on the fifth floor I was discharged. It was a formality for the treatment to begin. Similar to a voodoo rite.

A month later I was back at the Hypertension Clinic. In the examining room, the nurse took my blood pressure while I was lying down. It was 200/130. She took it again, 200/124, then it was 200/104. She then listened to my heart, read my chart and looked over all the medication I was taking to make certain they did not conflict with the blood-pressure pill. After she discussed it with the doctor, I received a prescription for Propronol, 10 mg. three times a day. Also Lasix, four mg. per day instead of the 2 mg. I had been taking.

We brought the prescription downstairs to the Pharmacy and waited. Stephanie got a headache from the heavy tobacco smoke that filled the waiting area and went out to the car while I remained for an hour and a half till the prescription was filled.

A week later we were back in the Hypertension Clinic. My pressure was 200/100 in sitting position and 185/95 in lying position. I weighed 140 pounds and got an increase in my Propronol, 20 mg. three times per day, and was told to continue with four mg. of Lasix per day.

From there I went to get my sore and creaking ankles X-rayed. After the usual hassle, I brought the film to the nurse in the Rheumatology Clinic. After a long wait Dr. C. called me into the room where a young female and male doctor were asked to diagnose me. Dr. C. asked me what I was doing now that I was not working. I told him I was chairperson of the Letters Committee of the Mullins Fine Arts Council and editor of their literary magazine, *High Tide*, plus many other activities. Then, on checking the X-ray films, he saw some deterioration in the small joints, although the ankle still looked good. After I got my blood drawn, Stephanie and I left.

Stephanie went with me to my next monthly appointment at the Hypertension Clinic. This time my pressure was a little lower, 180/96 in the sitting position and 175/96 while lying down. My pulse rate was also lower. Nurse said the lab test showed I was still anemic, so she prescribed iron for me. Also I was to continue on the same hypertension medication dosage.

Even with the drugs, my blood pressure was still elevated and I was still haunted by the thought that it was caused by something threatening, something that had not yet manifested itself.

In the meantime I continued my activities. The *High Tide* magazine had been put together one evening and, on the following morning, I drove to the printer in Devon and instructed him on what we wanted. On the way home I suddenly felt a nausea come over me. When I finally drove into my driveway, the nausea had almost overwhelmed me, and I was seized by a chill and severe weakness. I got out of my car and tried to vomit, but nothing but a little gas came up. I staggered into the house and phoned 911, and in a few minutes the police came with oxygen, and carried me on a stretcher to the ambulance and rushed me to the V.A. Hospital Emergency Room. In the Emergency Room, the E.K.G. turned out negative. My temperature was 102.8. They took blood and urine tests and found that I had a severe urinary infection.

I had a nurse notify Stephanie at her place of employment and she came down as soon as she could with a worried expression on her face. I told her it was nothing serious, just an infection in my kidneys. She relaxed, but only a little.

Stephanie and I were left alone in the examining room for quite a long time. I had to go to the bathroom, so I got off the table. But I was so weak that I was barely able to walk. It was only with Stephanie's help that I managed to get to the bathroom. She went inside with me despite someone warning her that she could "not go in there." After I had a fluid bowel movement, she helped me get back to the Emergency Room, where we continued waiting. I was thirsty, so Stephanie gave me a cup of water.

Finally, a couple of doctors arrived. I was transferred to a stretcher and sent to get my chest X-rayed. After that I was placed in a bed on the fifth floor. There a young doctor took my oral medical history, which he would compare with my medical charts when he read them, then he stuck an I.V. into my arm. An antibiotic, Amphacilin, was periodically injected into the line.

I was exhausted and wanted to get to sleep, but when the doctor finally left around 8:30 P.M. I was immediately sent to X-ray for I.V.P., kidney X-rays. It was after midnight before I was FINALLY back in my bed. It seems not to matter to the doctors and hospital staff how sick and exhausted a patient might be, they will perform their routine duties even if they have to do it over the patient's dead body.

The next morning, the doctor tried to push a tube into my nostril to get a sample of fluid from my stomach. But my stomach was so distended with air that I began to gag and heave up a lot of gas. This time, the nausea was greatly relieved and the doctor tried again and got the tube in with no difficulty.

Later I was sent down for another X-ray, a frontal view of my kidneys to check for stones.

In the morning I received a Tylenol suppository to help reduce my fever, but it gave me diarrhea. I called for a nurse, which proved futile. I got out of bed, grabbed my cane, but I could not find my goddamn slippers, so I walked barefooted quickly down the hallway toward the toilet pushing the pole on its little wheels with the two I.V. bottles jangling overhead and got to the bathroom just in time. Subsequently, I continued going to the bathroom all day long, some ten times, passing nothing but fluid stools. Yet my stomach remained bloated, it seemed locked in silence and would not pass gas.

The doctor told me it was because my stomach was rebelling against an infection in the stomach area. I told the doctor that I had passed no urine all day. He left to talk to other doctors about it.

I was transferred to the Medical Intensive Care Unit and

hooked up to the heart monitor, and to the wall pump to draw air and fluids from my stomach, yet my nausea and bloating persisted all day.

The next morning, my stomach was even worse. I was relieved a little when the doctor removed the uncomfortable tube from my nose. Because of the persistant nausea and belly distention, I had a very miserable day. I was given an anti-nausea pill (Compozine) which helped, but my stomach still remained bloated and the Compozine made me sleepy. Friends who came to visit me, including Stephanie, had to leave early because I kept dozing off on them.

My temperature was dropping and my diarrhea had stopped, but, despite the enormous amounts of urine I was finally passing, the kidneys were not filtering out the toxins that were building up in my bloodstream. Doctors believed it was only a temporary kidney failure. Because I myself felt certain it was only temporary, I was not worried.

I remained bloated and nauseous, and was on a liquid diet which I was unable to completely consume.

Finally on the fourth day, doctors told me my kidneys were beginning to function again. I was put on a full liquid diet and had a bowl of farina which was delicious and satisfying. My belly was still distended, a cough I had picked up in M.I.C.U. was still with me and X-rays showed that my hip joints were still free of infection.

Doctors said I was doing much better now and I was transferred back to the ward.

The next day the I.V. was removed from my arm and I was free to get around much better. My appetite was bad and, when the supper tray arrived, I drank only the apple juice from it. My stomach felt bad all evening. I had a strong urge for tomato juice and I remembered the therapeutic effect it once had on my stomach. Stephanie and I went to the Canteen, but the vending machines were all out of tomato juice.

Therefore, I settled for tomato soup which I heated in the micro-wave oven. From there on my stomach felt good.

Later I told the dietician about the tomato juice and, when the dinner tray arrived, I got two bowls of tomato soup, one cup of tomato juice, two strawberry shakes and coffee with milk and sugar. My stomach felt good.

Doctors told me I was doing well and the next day I would get more I.V.P. kidney X-rays to see if the stones were passed. The doctor said I would get an I.V. first, to make me more hydrated so that the dye that would go into the kidneys would not be too highly concentrated. This was to ensure that the kidneys, which were beginning to function, would not be slowed down with the test.

After supper the doctor put the I.V. into my arm in preparation for tomorrow's I.V.P. Before bedtime I received Citrus of Magnesium.

In the morning, after getting two enemas, I was in X-ray. When the ordeal was completed I was told to return in an hour, which I did, and six more exposures were made from two angles, to see how the dye had moved. Then I was told to return in the afternoon, at which time they took one more exposure.

I phoned Stephanie to bring my clothes so that I could go on a weekend pass. I was eating supper when she arrived and we were both in a happy and humorous mood. At this point the doctor came in and said the overall decision by the doctors was that it was best for me that they cancel the leave of absence. Though I was improving steadily, I was not yet fully recovered, he said. This was a critical point in my recovery and it was best for me to be here for them to watch if I got the actual symptoms.

Greatly disappointed, I reluctantly accepted his opinion. Stephanie was sad and she came to visit me all day on the Saturday and Sunday I had to stay in the dreary hospital. No doctors made their rounds and the hospital staff was reduced to a minimum.

On Monday morning, the doctors made their rounds. They would first stop just outside the patient's door and mumble to each other, filling each other in on the latest condition of the patient. Then they would come in and talk to the patient. They expressed their opinion that they believed my fever was due to the partial obstruction in my right kidney, where it was difficult for antibiotics to get at. They were keeping their eye on it to see what would happen, perhaps the obstruction might clear up on its own accord.

A young specialist from Disease Control came to question and examine me to try to determine the reason for my lingering fever. Later he returned with three of his colleagues and I was asked more questions.

Gradually, over the days, my appetite kept increasing and my stomach was less bothered with nausea. My doctor told me I was doing fine, my kidneys were working and I would be "going home soon." My diet had been changed from low to high sodium.

In the morning, I got up feeling good, no nausea or diarrhea. For breakfast I had ham and eggs, oatmeal, tomato juice, toast and butter and coffee. And I felt very good after eating every bit of it, and I was raring to go on the weekend pass the doctors had promised me.

When the doctors came on their morning rounds all my hopes for the weekend pass were dashed to pieces. The head of the group of doctors did not like the idea of my going home on a weekend pass. He seemed nervous and abrupt and added that things were still a little "too rocky." I asked him what he meant by rocky. He said my temperature was still up. I pointed out to him that my temperature was normal all week without any fever. He was annoyed and said it was in my best interest that I remain in the hospital, and he abruptly left with the rest of the doctors, except the intern who had been treating me on a regular basis. He said we would talk about it later, then ran off to catch up with the group.

When he returned he explained that they had found A-typical cells in my urine, which indicated a growth of some kind rather than a stone. They did not know whether it was benign or malignant. I sat there stunned and sickened by this news. A few minutes ago I felt as fit as a Stradivarius, now I felt like an old busted-up fiddle.

Regardless of my devastation, I still had my heart set on going home for the weekend. All right, I reasoned, so I have some kind of growth in my kidney. Still, what would be the difference between my staying here in the dreary hospital and spending the weekend at home? The only difference I could see was that I would be more miserable here than I would be at home. Therefore I immediately left my room and went out into the hallway in search of my doctor. After I found him I explained to him my feelings about it. He agreed with me, but had to talk to the other doctors.

After talking to a urologist, he said they okayed my weekend pass. Despite the great unknown danger hanging over my head, I was relieved that I was told the truth. It was easier to face my problems when I knew exactly what I had to deal with, and I was especially delighted to be going home where Stephanie and I would maintain an optimistic outlook as we had always done. As for the kidney growth, we would cross that bridge when we came to it.

Chapter 5

When I returned from my weekend pass, the doctor told me I would be transferred to the Urology Ward, but they would continue to follow me up.

After I was transferred to 3E, the urologist told me I would be getting a cystoscopic examination and more I.V.P. X-rays to check the kidney further.

In the evening, I received a liquid diet, then Castor Oil for the upcoming I.V.P.

On the following morning, I was in the X-ray room where exposures were made with the X-ray head rotating over my kidneys. Then a doctor injected the dye, and many more lamination X-rays were made.

Back in my room I busied myself reading a book while anxiously waiting for the doctors to give me the results. A few hours later, I learned that all the doctors had left for the day. How in hell can they be so goddamn heartless? I asked myself. They promised me that they would tell me as soon as they had received the results. "Goddamn, self-serving assholes," I said angrily in low tones.

I asked an amiable male nurse who was on duty if he would do me a favor and look at my chart to let me know the results of my kidney X-rays.

At first he was reluctant to do it, but when I explained the situation to him, he agreed.

When he returned, he told me the doctor would be able to

better explain the results to me in the morning. But one thing he was sure of, it was not as serious as they had suspected. Although I was slightly relieved, I was still worried over what exactly they had found.

In the morning my doctor, a wholesome-looking boy-next-door type with a pink cherubic face, whose name was Bobby O'N., happily told me he had "good news." The left kidney, which was not functioning at all, and the right kidney which had the partial blockage, were now both working well. The X-rays revealed nothing in terms of a growth. They would study it further with cytology tests to see if there were still any suspicious cells in the urine. They would also continue the blood tests to keep an eye on how well the kidneys were working.

At dinner time I received a low-sodium diet, just the opposite of what the doctor had ordered. He wanted me to take in more salt in order for me to retain more fluid. My kidneys were putting out more fluid than I was taking in, despite the enormous amounts of water I drank.

My doctors from the fifth floor came to see me. They were checking to learn if there were still any suspicious cells. If there were, they would want to know which kidney they were coming from. If a kidney had to be taken out, hopefully it would be the left one which was not functioning very well.

After I returned from a weekend pass, every patient got his breakfast tray except me. Chaos and confusion were still the hospital's most important product. After the usual hassle, I finally received my breakfast, which was cold. In the meantime Dr. O'N. put me on a twenty-four-hour urine collection.

In the afternoon I had another Cystoscopy. This time, to determine which kidney was exuding the abnormal cells, Dr. O'N. took a drain from each kidney. Not much urine came from the left one, I heard him say. Then he injected dye directly into each kidney while a young woman took X-rays.

It was a harrowing and uncomfortable experience that seemed to last forever.

Dr. O'N. later came to my room to say I could go home that day. The tests and X-rays did not reveal anything.

Getting discharged from the hospital was always a delightful moment for me and for Stephanie, who had arrived to pick me up. But we had to wait around for more than an hour before the papers were signed. It was exasperating, the way this place kept patients waiting needlessly. The hospital was overcrowded and the quality of service continued to decline. In the urology ward the rooms were built to accommodate one bed, but they were now jammed up with two beds. The ward was dirty, with an unhealthy environment, and I had acquired a chronic cough that cleared up only after I was discharged from the hospital. Plastic urinals were emptied, but never rinsed out, causing them to ferment so that the rooms smelled of rancid urine. Also, when the patients' water pitchers were filled with ice, stagnant water that sat in the sink's plumbing was added, giving the drinking water a putrid metallic taste.

Anyway, I was discharged from the sickening environment, at least for a little while.

A couple of weeks later, I was back in the hospital at Dr. O'N.'s request. The hospital was even more crowded than it had been, and there was a long waiting list of veterans waiting for a bed to become available. Apparently, unemployment during the 1976 recession had caused many to lose their medical insurance, as some of the new patients had told me, and they were forced to resort to the V.A. hospital, where they otherwise would have gone to other hospitals.

Dr. O'N. told me they would do some more blood work on me, and would start with an electrocardiogram. I asked him if there was anything wrong with my heart. He said no, it was just to check it for possible kidney surgery.

I was so astounded by the sound of "surgery" that I suddenly became stupified. But I recovered my speech soon enough to ask him the reason for this sudden talk of possible surgery.

He told me they had found a dark spot in my right kidney which they have not yet been able to identify.

"Could the spot in my kidney possibly be sludge from the infection and could this sludge be producing those bizarre cells?" I asked hopefully.

"That's possible," he said. "Also the infection could be producing them." I reconciled myself to the knowledge that these could be more likely possibilities for those cells than a tumor.

After returning from another weekend pass, I had to go through the same Cystoscopic ordeal. Dr. O'N. ran a probe into my right kidney and another in the left one, and drew out urine from each. They then ran dye into each and took a number of retrograde X-rays. It was a long drawn out process that lasted for two harrowing hours.

Later Dr. O'N. brought the X-ray films to my room to show me the results. One from the lamination series showed the kidneys very faintly because the kidneys were not working fully and therefore did not absorb the dye properly. It was not till Dr. O'N. took the retrograde X-rays that we were able to see the golf-club-head shaped object about two inches in length. Then he showed me the X-rays he had taken that day. The same object was clearly visible, but this time it was turned 180 degrees in the opposite direction. Dr. O'N. was puzzled by it. It was obvious that it was floating, which precluded it being a tumor, which would have been rooted. He said it might be a stone or some kind of glob left over from the infection.

The following morning, I was in the Nuclear Medicine room on the second floor, lying on a wicker bed, under a gamma-ray camera. The technician who injected the radioactive fluid into my arm was clumsy and careless. Without bothering to look at the veins to see which would be best to inject, he simply jabbed the needle into a vein at random. Then he began mumbling about having problems and playing with the needle trying to get it into the center of the vein. When he finally injected the fluid, I asked him if it had gone into the vein. He said, "Some of it did," and proceeded on with the test nonchalantly. I was astonished by his indifference to what he was doing. Most of the hospital staff were well trained and highly skilled individuals. Yet lately, it seemed to me, I had been seeing more people giving tests to patients with either little training or total incompetence. It was clear to me why there were so many malpractice suits in this country. It was simply because there was a hell of a lot of malpractice!

Anyway, he took a series of fifteen gamma photos timed at certain intervals, and the test was over. How accurate the test was was anyone's guess.

Later Dr. O'N. and his partner, Dr. B., a tall black man wearing steel-rimmed glasses, came to my room to tell me that my original urologist from 1961 had looked at the X-rays and believed the object in question was a stone. Dr. O'N. said they would wait for the Cytology report on the cells and the radioactive scan. (The scan turned out to be useless.) Then, he said, regardless of what the cells looked like, I would be able to go home. He would send the cells to another pathologist for another opinion. Then in about a month, he would have me come back to be checked just to be sure.

The next morning, Dr. O'N. said he had another doctor look at my X-rays, and he too thought it was a stone, but he suggested that it should be removed. If not, it could cause blockage and create problems that would seriously damage the right kidney, the only good kidney I had left. Although the right kidney was chronically infected, as long as it remained open with urine allowed to flow freely, the bacteria were kept under control. However, if the stone should block the urine, the bacteria would breed into a full-blown infection, like the one I had in June. If the object was just a spongy mass, it could eventually disintegrate.

Dr. O'N. said I could go home, but he wanted me to return Friday morning so he could give me the results of the tests.

Friday morning Stephanie and I returned to the hospital and waited from 9 A.M. to 11 A.M. before Dr. O'N. and Dr. B. came into the room. Dr. O'N. repeated the scenario about the need for the stone to come out. The test from the pathologist had come back negative, which was quite a relief to Stephanie and me. We thanked him and immediately left.

I returned on Monday and Dr. O'N. said he was going to do another Cystoscopy on me to see if the stone had moved or if it might be sludge, but he got tied up with an emergency operation, so the test was cancelled.

Later Dr. O'N. returned to my room, still wearing his green operating clothes, and apologized for not being able to do the test. He said he had talked to an anesthesiologist who assured him he could put me in a semiconscious condition that would allow me to breath on my own during the surgery, therefore avoiding the tracheotomy.

In the afternoon, I was back in the dreaded Cysto room. I had retrograde X-rays done on my right kidney. Dr. O'N. said the "thing" was still there. Then he told me he would schedule my surgery for tomorrow. I was shocked by this, because up to now we were only talking about the surgery. Now suddenly it had become a harsh reality.

He also added that, if he found a tumor, it would be best to remove the entire kidney. Removing only the tumor would be no guarantee that it would not grow back, and a second operation would be even worse. But the decision was up to me.

I looked at the last X-ray, and saw that the object now had a different shape, and it appeared to have branches radiating from it.

To lose the only good kidney I had was not an easy decision for me to make. I painfully pondered over it and finally agreed with Dr. O'N. that, if a tumor was found, it would be best to remove the entire kidney.

I already knew, from past experience, that if the tumor turned out to be malignant, even the removal of the entire kidney gave no survival guarantees. A friend of mine had a kidney removed because of a malignant tumor and he had died in six months. Therefore I was very much aware of what I was possibly facing. Yet I was far from taking any defeatist attitude. I still clung to my optimism because I felt the odds were on my side. From all the X-rays I had seen, I was almost certain that the object was a stone. But even if it should turn out to be a tumor, there was still a fifty-fifty chance that it would be benign.

Later, an Oriental anesthesiologist came to see me. He said he was eighty percent sure he could get a breathing tube into my windpipe, I was pleased to hear that and told him I was scheduled for surgery the next day. He looked at his list and said I was not on it. Familiar with the sloppy interdepartmental communications in the hospital, I was not too surprised. But I hoped it would be straightened out before I got to the operating room.

The nurse sent me to the "Prep" room to get shaved. On the way over, I met the anesthesiologist and told him I was on my way to the Prep Room. He inquired at the nurses' station and was told that indeed I was going to surgery tomorrow. They had crossed someone's name off the list and added mine.

After getting the shave, I returned to my room.

Just before supper, Dr. O'N. came in and said they all agreed that the stone should come out. They were ninety percent sure it was a stone. I was somewhat consoled by the fact that at least the odds were on my side. I told him about my massive bleeding during my hip operation. He said my blood chemistry was good so he did not foresee any bleeding problem. He said the operation would take about one and a half hours, if everything went well.

A nurse gave me an antibiotic injection which felt like a bee sting.

At bedtime I received an injection. "To help you sleep," the nurse said.

The next morning I was up at 6 A.M. for another antibiotic injection, and was prepared for surgery. Dr. O'N. came in to tell me that he was almost certain the anesthesiologist would be able to ventilate me. If not, they would have someone there ready to do the "trac."

At 10 A.M. I received another antibiotic injection, and an I.V. to hydrate me.

A half an hour later Stephanie came in and tried to cheer me up, which she did. Yet though she did not let on, I could detect that she herself was worried. She remained with me till I was wheeled out on a stretcher.

In the operating room, the anesthesiologist sprayed my throat with a numbing substance, slowly working the hard plastic tube into my throat, adding more spray as he went in at deeper levels. But it did not go in all the way, so he slipped a tube into my right nostril with perfect ease and no discomfort to me. I was breathing easily through the tube and I heard someone say, "It's right on the money." After that I knew nothing until I woke up in the recovery room.

As I was regaining consciousness, I thought I was still in the operating room and the surgery had not yet begun. A moderate pain in my right side convinced me that the surgery had indeed been done.

I asked the nurse in the recovery room how it went. She told me with a smile that they had removed a stone and my kidney was still in. Although I was barely conscious, I was elated by this happy news. Then Stephanie came into the recovery room to see me. She was all smiles.

From the recovery room I was moved to the ward, this time in a private room with only one bed. I felt very sleepy and told Stephanie that it would be best if she went home, and I spent most of that day and night sleeping. That evening Stephanie returned and my brother Joe and his wife Irene also dropped in. I carried on my end of the conversation all right, but I kept dozing off for a minute or two in between. Right after they left, I immediately fell into a deep sleep.

In the morning, Dr. B. came in to change the bandage. I still had a tube in the incision attached to a plastic bag into which some blood had drained. I inquired about it, and Dr. B. said it was to allow the blood to drain from around my kidney rather than accumulate into a pool that could possibly cause infection. I asked him who did the surgery. He said he did.

I received pancakes and syrup for breakfast which I ate slowly.

Dr. O'N. came in and showed me the stone they had removed. It was an irregularly-shaped pink stone almost two inches long and resembled a tropical sea coral. He said the stone was a time bomb. If it had gotten any bigger it would have blocked off the whole kidney. He said everything went smoothly and felt my belly, which was very distended. He was surprisd that they had given me a regular breakfast. I should have been on a liquid diet for at least twenty-four hours. At his request, a nurse gave me a suppository to help me pass gas, but it did not work.

Two nurses helped me out of bed and walked me and my I.V. pole down the hall. I felt weak and stiff. When I was returned to bed, I fell asleep until dinner came. It consisted of clear soup and tea.

Around 3 P.M. they got me up again and walked me to the end of the hall and back. Then later, I walked alone all the way to Intensive Care and back.

I complained to Dr. O'N. about my terrible stomach discomfort. He told me not to eat or drink anything at all. The I.V. I still had was providing me with plenty of fluids.

In the evening I began passing some gas and felt much better and my stomach was less distended. The next morning, Dr. L., the anesthesiologist, came to see me. I told him he had done a very good job getting the breathing tube into my windpipe. He smiled broadly and said I was a good patient.

In the afternoon I received one unit of blood to make up for the slight deficit I had.

The next day, Dr. O'N. ordered another unit of blood. The male nurse, after several unsuccessful efforts to get the I.V. needle into my vein, gave up, and came back with a doctor who finally put it in.

When the plastic bag was almost half empty, the blood stopped flowing through the tube. I put on the call light and kept blinking it to attract a nurse. After a half hour, as the blood stagnated in the tube, I yelled for the nurse as loud as I could. For a long time no one responded.

Eventually, a male orderly, who always seemed to be in a trance, came into my room. He fumbled around with the little clamps on the tubing and accomplished nothing. Yet he continued fumbling with it and made it even worse by filling the line with air. I told him to leave it alone and to go get the nurse. In his flat voice, he said the nurse was in another building on an emergency, but he would go get her.

Twenty minutes later, the nurse arrived and expertly got the air out and the blood flowing properly again. I asked her whether the blood would coagulate by standing like that for almost an hour. She said, "No, it was protected in the tubing. Sometimes it took up to five hours to give to some patients who needed it given at a slow pace."

The anxiety I had been going through was now dispelled by the nurse who, working the ward all alone and obviously overworked, still maintained her empathy with the patients.

When the big, spaced-out orderly returned to take my vital signs, he said, "You got blood yesterday, didn't it stop on you?"

"Yes," I said, "but when the nurse came, it was straightened out." Still a bit angry I resentfully added, "I just don't see why in hell they can't have more nurses on duty. Instead, they put a guy like you in charge." This statement did not seem to faze him in the least. His graying blond hair was neatly combed and his white uniform was immaculate, and in his spooky, robot-like trance he continued making his rounds with his shoulders held back and his spine, which was normal, held poker straight as though he were ready to participate in a military parade. Very weird. I mean, for a guy like that to be left in charge of post-operative patients! Yet I could not help feeling sorry for this individual who, for all I knew, might be a very lonely and broken-hearted person. Later, when he returned to my room, I apologized to him for having spoken so rudely to him. He said, "Oh, that was all right."

As the days passed, I continued to improve. My clear liquid diet went to solid liquid, then to normal diet, and the long drainage tube and the plastic bag were removed, as well as the I.V. Now all that I had in me was a small drain tube and stitches covered over with a small bandage.

The head nurse, a pretty dark-haired New Yorker, told me

I was doing amazingly well. Yet for some inexplicable reason, I was feeling uptight and apprehensive. This depression had begun about an hour earlier when I had a slight fever of 100.1 degrees and was cautioned by the nurse that I should avoid pneumonia by breathing deeply and coughing frequently. Although that contributed something to my worry, it was actually my elevated blood pressure of 190/116 that brought on the bulk of my concern. The blood pressure continued to remain elevated, and I found it impossible to relax. My mind was crowded with visions of having my kidneys removed because of high blood pressure.

Finding it impossible to tolerate further my internal agitation, I asked for a Valium. The nurse gave me 10 mg. of it, and I slept soundly the rest of the night.

I got up in the morning feeling relaxed and rested. The occasional minor pain in my right side was completely gone. I got out of bed without any assistance. My temperature was 98 degrees, my pulse was 64, and my blood pressure was 150/82. My urine, which had red blood in it due to the surgery, was now "perfectly clear" as Tricky Nixon would say.

Every morning since I had been on solid foods, I craved for some eggs, which I ascertained would be very nutritious for me. But for the past six days, all I had received for breakfast was either bad-tasting pancakes or French Toast, with the trays constantly loaded with sugary junk foods. I wondered how it was possible for a patient to recover on that kind of sickening diet. Breakfast was the only meal I was able to actually eat fully.

Anyway, I had Stephanie bring in some C and E vitamins. I felt that I needed all the help I could get.

The dietician was surprised when I told her I had not had a single egg since my surgery, and she assured me that she would straighten that out.

The small drainage tube had been removed a few days earlier, and Dr. O'N. now removed the stitches and told me I would get discharged on Saturday. As I realized that I would have to wait two more days before my discharge, I said, "How about making it Friday?"

He thought about it for a moment, then said, "Okay, you talked me into it."

I liked Dr. O'N. He was not pompous or secretive about his profession as so many doctors were. He and I had a good rapport and worked together as a team, and had a healthy respect for each other.

For my next breakfast I finally received scrambled eggs!

Dr. O'N. told me I could leave at 10 A.M. He cautioned me to take it easy, to do nothing strenuous for at least three weeks.

Stephanie picked me up, and away we went.

At my next clinic appointment, Stephanie stayed home from work to go with me to Renal Clinic in Building Two. My blood pressure was high, I gave a urine sample, and I weighed 140 pounds. I had always considered arthritis as being my principle impediment. Now it suddenly occurred to me that my kidneys, which were related to my high blood pressure, were a new addition to my woes.

Three weeks later, instead of my going to the Clinic, Dr. O'N. wanted me to be admitted for a few more tests. After the usual long hassle, I was finally admitted and was placed in the same room I was in the last time. Dr. O'N. explained that, due to the Thanksgiving holiday, the X-ray staff would do only emergency X-rays. Since mine was not an emergency, he suggested I go home on a weekend pass and return Monday morning. I told him that on Mondays I was teaching American Labor History at the University of Bridgeport's alternative program and would rather come in on Tuesday morning. He said it was all right.

On returning to the hospital, I had my kidneys X-rayed. In the afternoon Dr. O'N. told me the X-rays looked all right, and added that the stone they had removed from my kidney was caused by uric acid. They wanted more urine samples to determine how much uric acid was being secreted. Then they would prescribe medication that would cut down the uric acid.

In the evening I was discharged from the hospital.

On Friday, Stephanie and I returned to the hospital to pick up a gallon jug for a twenty-four-hour urine collection. Also, I left a fresh sterile urine sample. Dr. O'N. said he had talked to other doctors at the hospital who suggested that it would be best if I did not get sulfa pills which would completely eliminate the E-Coli bacteria. Because of the stones, this would not prevent further infections. The E-Coli had established residence in the stone areas, and in effect kept other bacteria from getting a foothold. The other bacteria could possibly be more virulent forms that might be harder or impossible to treat.

At my next Renal Clinic appointment, I received a prescription for Allopurinol to keep the uric acid down and prevent further stone formation. I now weighed 142 pounds.

In the meantime, while I was campaigning for a city office, my left hip began transmitting sporadic sharp pains through the front of my thigh at certain movements. Dr. R., the surgeon who had put my artificial hip joints in, later verified through X-rays that the glue that held them in was breaking down.

In May of 1977, on one of my Renal Clinic appointments, the doctor in charge asked me if I would like to volunteer for a test being conducted at a major local hospital. He introduced me to a young bearded intern who explained that the experiment was being done to discover the sugar utilization of persons with kidney problems. Kidney patients have more strokes and heart attacks than normal. They suspected that, due to kidney damage, the sugar was not utilized properly, resulting in arterial deterioration. He asked me if I would like to participate in the test. It would be from 8 A.M. to 1 P.M., and I would be paid $50.00 for my troubles. If this would help medical knowledge, and possibly myself, and since it would not be harmful to me, I told him that I would do it. The intern took my name, address and phone number and said he would call me.

About a week later, I got a call from the bearded intern who told me to report to the hospital at 8 A.M. He also told me not to take any Inderol that night and not to eat anything in the morning, but it would be all right to take my Lasix, Indocin and Allopurinol.

At the hospital, on the fifth floor, a doctor in his 40's and the intern were working on a couple of other renal patients. After getting weighed, I sat in a chair, and the intern began putting the I.V. into my arm. As he struggled to get the needles in, there was a lot of fumbling and nose-blowing into a handkerchief (he had a bad cold). At one point in the process, he almost fell as he tripped over a wastebasket, and he did not in the least bit inspire me with confidence. When he finally finished putting bandages over the needles, the two needles caused me a lot of discomfort.

I complained about the pain and the older doctor came over to look at it and immediately unraveled the bulky bandages, rearranged the needles, and bandaged them neatly. My arm was then free of pain.

While the fluid was slowly trickling into my veins, I sat there prepared to pass the time by reading. But gradually a chill came over me. I put my jacket over my shoulders and continued reading. Yet the chilliness persisted, my hands were ice cold and I began to tremble. At this point I was moved to a smaller room where another patient was lying on a bed. I was seated beside a control mechanism and another line was attached to my I.V. which was for insulin.

I complained about feeling cold, and they put my hand in an electric warmer which brought heat to my hand, but it did nothing for the rest of my shivering body. Thinking it would pass, I tried to keep my mind off it as much as possible, hoping to hold out until the test was completed. But it was no use. The coldness continued increasing and my shivering became uncontrollable. The older doctor became very concerned when I told him I was feeling nauseous. He immediately drew a blood sample, I gave him a urine sample, and he rushed them to the lab. Then he phoned the V.A. hospital and I asked him to call Stephanie to let her know where I would be. Then they unhooked the insulin line and left the glucose line in until I was ready to leave. Finally, I was taken down in the elevator, by the intern, in a wheelchair and we waited in the lobby as the older doctor pulled up in his car. I got out of the wheelchair, climbed into the car and then, using the turnpike, we headed for the V.A. The doctor told me he did not think the test had anything to do with my sudden illness, and that I was probably already coming down with something.

In the Emergency Room, I had an I.V. put in, blood drawn again, and an E.K.G. My blood pressure was 185/113, and my temperature was 103.4 degrees.

After being interviewed by an intern and two doctors, I was taken out on a stretcher to X-ray. There was a long wait in X-ray and I was very thirsty, but when I asked for water I was told I was not allowed any water because of doctor's orders. I had my chest and abdomen X-rayed, then I was left in the hallway for quite a long time. When an escort finally brought me back to Emergency, I was kept lying on the stretcher in the hallway for more waiting. I kept asking for water, but was constantly refused. I was no longer shivering with cold, instead I was now burning up with fever, feeling weak and helpless and wondering who was the moronic doctor who had restricted my water. Everyone I asked told me the doctor was not available. Therefore there was no way I could talk to him about my kidney problems, and his subordinates were only following his iron dictum. How in hell did I get into this goddamn mess, I thought. This morning I got up feeling healthy as a frisky race horse and a few hours later I felt as though I were on the verge of death.

After convincing the intern that I needed the water to keep my kidneys open, he compromised his orders by giving me ice chips. I felt better almost immediately. Then he gave me a big cup of water to drink and I began to feel greatly improved. All I needed was water to drink! But I was in the clutches of doctors who not only did not bother to read my chart, but who also did not even confide in me. I knew absolutely nothing about the doctor's order that restricted me from drinking anything, that is not until the doctor was gone and lost forever.

At last, after four and a half hours of "emergency" treatment that almost killed me, I was brought to the ward on the fifth floor.

Outside of my chronic urinary tract infection, all the other tests they gave me proved negative. I was getting Amphicilin for the infection.

That night I woke from a deep sleep to find my bed covered with blood. The I.V. tube had pulled lose from its plug near the needle in my arm, and my blood was pouring out. There was also water all over the bed and floor that had leaked out of the glucose bottle. I immediately put on the call light.

The nurse changed the bottle and attached a new tube line. She did not think the tube was parted for very long, otherwise there would have been a lot more blood and water spilled.

She said that patients were sometimes found with their lines parted, when the nurse would notice a large pool of blood and water on the floor. I did not ask, but I wondered how many patients may have been found dead when that happened. In my opinion, I believe I.V. connections should have some kind of locking system to prevent them from accidently being pulled out while the patient slept.

More and more I found myself dreading to be in the hospital—a hospital was no place for sick people—and I yearned to get back home again where I was relatively safe from harm.

On the fourth day after being admitted, the doctors told me I was looking good and my chart confirmed it. And I felt good. They said that, despite all the tests, they were unable to trace the source of my sudden illness. But one of them said that, once in a million, an I.V. mixture could contain some substance that could cause such a reaction.

Then on that afternoon I was picked up by Stephanie and happily left on a discharge.

Chapter 6

At home, I recuperated very rapidly and, within days, I resumed my activity in the Independent Consumers Party, which was running a slate of candidates for city offices. I was not only one of the candidates but also the party's coordinator, press agent, and writer of the party's position papers. At the same time, my small book, titled *Brass Tacks*, had just been published and I was on TV promoting it; I was teaching American Labor History one day a week, and chairing the monthly meetings of the Letters Committee of the Mullins Fine Arts Council. I was quite busy and my health was perking along without problems.

Then abruptly, I was cut off from everything. One evening, after returning from a hectic meeting at which wine and cheese were served, I went to bed bloated and I kept waking up with severe burning sensations in my esophagus, which I tried to relieve with many spoonsful of antacids. On the following morning, I passed pitch-black stools mixed with red blood. I phoned Stephanie at her place of employment and had two more such bowel movements.

Stephanie drove me to the V.A. Emergency Room. This was on September 22, 1977, and I was returning into the clutches of the ponderous hospital where nightmares were for real.

I was weak, nauseous, light-headed and only slightly frightened because I knew what was happening from previous stomach bleedings. The nurse directed us to one of the rooms where she took my blood pressure, temperature and urine sample and told us to wait until the doctor could see me.

After some twenty minutes, a smiling young woman came in, introducing herself as Dr. F. I was surprised by her youthfulness. "You look like a high school student," I said, with a smile.

She laughed, "That's only my disguise."

When she studied my chart and asked me questions I could see in her a sort of solidity and confidence that comes from knowing one's profession.

"Your hematocrit indicates that you had lost a lot of blood," she said. "What kind of medication are you on?"

"I take four Indocin capsules and about fifteen to twenty aspirins a day, depending on how I feel."

"Do you take them with your meals?" she asked.

"Now I do. But it was only recently that a doctor told me about it. That's only after I lost most of my stomach lining."

"I'm sorry," was all she said.

A touch of anger came over me, and I said, "Most doctors don't have time to tell their patients how to take their medication."

She remained silent. I learned later that doctors never talk to patients about their colleagues.

I was brought into the Intensive Care Unit where I had ice water treatments that were of short duration. Since I had been through these treatments twice before I never felt in danger of dying.

The bleeding would stop for hours only to resume again and the ice water treatment would follow again.

During one of these treatments Big Ed Altieri, our flamboyant candidate for Mayor, came to visit me. He looked subdued and uneasy. He shook my hand with his large paw.

"How ya' doin', Mike?" he said, trying to sound cheerful.

"Pretty good, Ed. Sit down and take the load off," I said, as the nurse continued withdrawing from my stomach the dark pink ice water that stubbornly refused to come up clear.

Since it was difficult for me to speak at the time, Big Ed just sat there watching the ritual with a pained, hangdog expression on his ruddy and course face.

When the syringefuls began to appear almost red, I winced and shook my head slightly.

Looking ill, Big Ed got up, grabbed my hand briefly and immediately left.

A few minutes later the red turned pink and finally clear, eliciting a great sigh of relief from the nurse and me.

The next day berium X-rays revealed that I had a large duodenal ulcer.

On the third day I was no longer bleeding and was transferred to the ward in a room with three other patients, and given Citric of Magnesia to drink to clean out the berium from my stomach.

A while later I rushed to the bathroom and passed a lot of fluid. But when I got up to look at it, expecting to see a bowl full of white berium, I was shocked to see that it was full of red blood. I called the nurse to look at it and she confirmed that it was a lot of blood.

More blood was drawn from my arm for the hematocrit test, and I.V. was again put into my arm and a tube was again pushed into my nose down to my stomach. The syringe again drew out red blood and I was back to square one. Ruefully I surmised that it was the irritating laxative that had brought on this relapse, and anger flared up in me because of the crudeness of tests that do more harm than good for patients.

I received two more units of whole blood, and I was still left in the ward.

Gradually the stools turned back to normal. The syringe drew out of my stomach only clear ice water and I was greatly soothed when the tube and I.V. were removed.

It was wonderful being free of bleeding and being out of bed and feeling in a very good mood.

One of the patients had been discharged and the two other patients in my room were delighted to see me feeling better. We joked around, talked about generalities and then about politics. All three of us had diverse opinions and it became a lively and friendly exchange of ideas that lasted for quite some time, and I was enjoying it tremendously.

Suddenly a veil of fatigue descended upon me, bringing me to the edge of collapse, and I became abruptly silent. I went to my bed and laid down. A strange irritating discomfort that bordered on nausea invaded my insides, and the dreadful realization that I was bleeding again hit me like a freight train. I cursed myself for overexerting myself during my weakened condition.

The following morning I passed red stools. A blood test showed great loss of blood and my blood pressure was 90/60. Dr. F. again put an I.V. into my arm, then slid a tube into my nose and down to my stomach. Finally she pushed ice water into my stomach, withdrew it and, to our surprise, saw that it was clear of blood. To my great consolation, she pulled out the tube and the I.V. "I lucked out again," I said with a smile.

I lay down on my bed and was just beginning to relax when a nurse told me I had to get to the third floor for a rectal examination. After expressing my annoyance I got up, took my cane and went to the place I was directed to.

After I removed my robe and lowered my pajama bottoms, the doctor asked me to kneel down and bend face-down over a strange looking short table. Then the head of the bed was lowered and I was draped over it with my bare bottom up high.

I could hear the doctor shuffling through the drawers, then he said, "I'll be right back." I heard him leave and the door close. In that embarrassing position, I waited patiently. A few minutes later I heard the doctor's footsteps and then he was rattling the door knob. He knocked and called to me to open the door. Weak and stiff from my arthritis I did not think I could get myself up from that awkward position. I cursed the dummy for locking himself out and struggled hard to get up. Only by exerting myself to the fullest was I able to succeed.

The doctor apologized, got me back into position, and gently inserted the instrument, at the same time opening the passageway with air by squeezing a rubber bulb, going deeper and deeper. He drew out the instrument and said he did not see anything of significance. Then he inserted a wider one, going in only a short distance. After that it was all over and it was all quite painless.

In the afternoon Dr. F. returned to tell me that they had decided that I should have an endoscopy test. This meant that an instrument would be pushed down my throat to my stomach for a visual examination. There was a small risk of restarting the bleeding, but it would pinpoint the exact source of my problem in case surgery was necessary.

I was in no mood for risktaking. I was exhausted and all I wanted to do was rest and give myself a chance to heal.

I argued against the endoscopy test especially since there was some risk.

But Dr. F.'s argument for the need of such a test was so compelling and persuasive that, like the fool I often am, I finally agreed to accept it and signed the consent form.

I was brought to the preparation room near the O.R. and, feeling like Socrates, was handed a cup of obnoxious-tasting chemical to gargle my throat with. Soon my whole mouth became numb. Then I got up on the table and, while one of the two nurses held my hand to give me comfort and reassurance, the doctor ran an enormously thick instrument down my throat, going deeper and deeper till he was able to see inside of my stomach. All this time I was on the edge of panic, fearing that my breathing would be interrupted and no one would know about it till it was too late. But the nurse, holding my hand and talking to me soothingly, managed to keep me under control.

The doctor continued manipulating the scope, pumping air in for better viewing and trying to push it through the duodenal. But the duodenal would not let the instrument through, so he gave up and pulled it out completely, to my great alleviation.

The doctor said he saw no bleeding in the part of the stomach he was able to see. I got off the table and thanked the kind and gentle nurse for the comfort she gave me through the whole ordeal. The doctor had pinpointed nothing and the test was worse than worthless.

I was pushed in a wheelchair back to my room and soon after that I was bleeding again.

As I was being wheeled back into the Intensive Care Unit, feeling devastated and choking with rage and frustration, I cursed myself and the damn fools for reopening my poor ulcer. Instead of letting me rest and heal, the doctors had this stupid mania for tampering and tampering.

When I was in bed in the Intensive Care Unit they placed the plugs on my chest to monitor my heart. I already had an intervenous line placed in my arm and a tube in my nose down to my stomach.

Dr. F. filled the large syringe with ice water from a pan held by a nurse and injected the cold water into my stomach. After a few moments she withdrew the water, which was now bright red with blood. She pushed in and withdrew syringe after syringe of ice water for what seemed like hours.

But my bleeding continued and the ice cold water treatment also continued, causing everything in the midsection of my body to feel like a solid block of ice. Even with all the blankets over me I was cold and shivered uncontrollably. Through my chattering I asked, "How much longer?" "Till the bleeding stops," the doctor answered. The expression on her usually smiling face was grim. I felt a tug at my heart as I realized that I was in deep trouble.

I thought of Stephanie, who had been sitting in the waiting room so long and had left at nightfall. I wanted very much to see her, hold her hand and to tell her for possibly the last time how much I loved her.

But she was out of my reach and I felt in my heart a throbbing ache of loss and unfulfillment.

No matter how badly things were going for me, I was still determined to hang on.

Determined as I was, the shivering and the extreme cold were overwhelming me and becoming unbearable. I asked the doctor to stop a while so I could warm up a little. But as she struggled with the syringe, she told me she could not stop, not till the bleeding stopped.

As I suffered the extreme cold, I tried to imagine myself lying on a hot sunny beach. But it did no good, my body just shivered unceasingly.

Working the syringe was hard work for the doctor and the nurse who kept switching places to spell each other. They were both exhausted but unflinching in their resolve to stop the bleeding.

I felt that I would freeze to death before they could stop the bleeding.

I was already visualizing the doctor's report: "Our efforts to stop the hemorrhage were successful. Unfortunately the patient succumbed to hypothermia."

My mind reeled. No, no, I won't let it happen. It's all a

horrible mistake! I just refuse to die on the grounds that it might kill me. I have been a rebel most of my life. I can beat this standing on my head. After all, I had already beaten a giant corporation. I had worked for the company for nine and a half years, first as a tool maker, then as an inspector, and I was also a union shop steward. I had written an article that was published in a New Haven newsletter criticizing union-company collusion, and I was subsequently fired. After a five-year legal free-speech and press battle, the Federal Court unanimously upheld a lower court's ruling that I should be awarded back pay and all legal expenses, setting a new legal precedent. Lawyers across the country agreed that this landmark decision could benefit all workers. In the face of impossible odds I had fought back and I had won. I won! I won!...damn, it's...it's cold, cold....

My eyesight and my mind grew dim and there were lapses in the activities around me. Many things slid past me unnoticed. Medical people appeared at my bedside who came and went. One moment there would be a new arrival, I would blink my eyes for what seemed like only a fraction of a second, and suddenly that person was no longer there. Everything around me was hazy and unreal.

I was slipping away. Yet, curiously enough, I felt no panic or fear. Instead, I felt a certain relief mixed with comfort, a sort of twilight zone between caring and not caring.

Suddenly I was jarred back to my senses by a sharp jabbing pain in my right ankle.

"What's happening?" I hysterically asked my doctor.

"The surgeon's making an incision to get a catheter into your vein," she answered calmly.

"Why?" I demanded.

"To try to run it to your duodenal to inject a medicine that may stop the bleeding."

I grimaced as the sharp, cutting pain moved to a new site

on my ankle. It was a hacking, pulling, pressing pain that was excruciating.

"What in hell's happening?" I sputtered through my clenched teeth.

"The first vein broke. He's trying another one."

I tried to ponder this but felt myself slipping back into my delirium. Everything around me, including my ankle pain, faded in and faded out.

Then I was running, I was running for the first time in a long time. I had discarded my cane and was running through a weed-covered field feeling free as the wind. Bursting with elation I was eager to get to my wife to tell her that I was well again. I ran into many obstacles and found myself in a large house going through many doors and getting nowhere. I was caught in a maze that was frustrating beyond endurance.

Finally I felt myself floating and saw the ceiling lights moving overhead as if on a conveyor. I was lying on a stretcher being pushed rapidly by several persons. "Where going?" I mumbled.

"O.R.," someone answered.

Being rushed toward the operating room was the last thing I was conscious of.

Sometime later I felt a glimmer of reality moving in on me. I heard someone tell me that the surgery was over. But I was so heavily sedated that I could not respond. I also learned that I was in the Postoperative Intensive Care ward. Intermittently I could hear people talking but could not comprehend anything that was being said. Most of the time there were long periods of complete unconsciousness.

Somehow I felt if I did not wake up I would surely die. I struggled to open my eyes, to try to say something to Stephanie who I knew was there at my bedside. But all I could manage was to open my eyes for a second and try to mumble something to her before going under again.

I was frightfully determined not to allow myself to fall into a coma from which I felt I would never recover. I fought and struggled incessantly to regain consciousness. But, like a drowning person, I merely popped up to the surface for a brief second, only to sink into darkness again and again.

Then I heard a nurse tell me that I must rest and must stop fighting the pain-killing drugs. After that, I rested more peacefully.

The next day I was more lucid. Stephanie was there with a smile on her face, we held hands and she said, "How do you feel, hon?"

"A little whoozy," I said.

"You look a lot better today," she said.

I was happy to see her, but I was not in a festive mood to demonstrate it.

"Were you here yesterday?" I asked.

"Yes, I was here all day."

"Did I say anything?"

"Yes. Everytime you woke up you said, 'I love you.' "

Although I had been struggling to tell her, for what I thought would be the last time, that I loved her, I was quite surprised to learn that I had actually succeeded in doing so.

After a brief pause, I said, "Hell, I didn't think I was getting through to you."

"You got through, loud and clear," she said, with a smile.

During a considerable pause, her mood turned somber.

Then she told me about the nightmare she had the night I went to surgery.

"I saw a lot of people around your bed and a doctor was cutting and cutting into your leg and trying to push a tube in your vein. It was lasting a long time and I could see that you were in a lot of pain. It was too much for me to watch, I could not stand it any longer so I yelled at the doctor, 'Stop it! Stop it!, please! No more! That's enough!' Then I woke up and suddenly sat up. I turned on the light and looked around and said, 'Oh my God! He's going to surgery!' It was three o'clock in the morning and I couldn't sleep any more. It was so real I couldn't get it out of my mind! Then, after a while, the phone rang. It was the doctor telling me that they took you to surgery. I said, 'I know.' Then I asked him how you were, and he said you were all right."

She stopped and looked down at her hands meditatively. She had described the scene so accurately that I felt a chill run up my spine. It was incredible! I thought. An event that defied all logic had actually transpired! I believed in the possibility of extrasensory perception, but what she described went way beyond the pale of psychic phenomena, something I had always been skeptical about. Could they both be one and the same? I wondered.

We were both silent for a long time. Then my mind was diverted to my stomach, which was quite painful, and I asked Stephanie if she knew how much of my stomach was removed.

"I don't know," she said. "Nobody told me anything."

I called one of the nurses over and asked her. She said they had removed more than half of my stomach.

I remember in my semi-conscious periods hearing that I had lost part of my stomach, and I felt that it was only a small part of it, just enough to stop the hemorrhage. But the reason for removing more than half my stomach was something I did not understand.

A heavy drowsiness was descending over me and I kept drifting off. Each time I did, I fought back to stay awake.

Stephanie put her hand on mine, and said, "Don't fight it. Go back to sleep, you need all the rest you can get."

My eyes were closed and I wanted to tell her to go home and also get some rest. But being in a state of euphoria, I was unable to generate enough energy to verbally respond to her.

112 FOOTSTEPS TO SURVIVAL

All I could do was to gently squeeze her hand, and immediately fall asleep.

I woke up when a nurse was taking my blood pressure, after which she took down a nearly empty bottle from the I.V. pole and put in its place a full one, which fed me glucose, vitamins and intermittently my medication.

Stephanie was still there. This time I was able to say, "Hon, go home and get some rest."

She hesitated a moment, then said, "I want to stay here with you."

"But I'll be sleeping most of the time. There's no point in your sitting here all day."

She finally agreed and went home.

The next day I was a bit more conscious of my surroundings, but still having spells of drowsiness. In the afternoon Stephanie was back again and I was glad to see her. She brought me the mail and told me of the phone calls she got. My brothers Joe, Bill, Richard and one of my sisters, Dorothy, wanted to know how I was doing. Also Jack Fernandez, the black man who worked in an aircraft plant when I had worked there, wanted to know if there was anything he could do for us. Ever since I had been fired from my job he had been helping me in many different ways. He would drive me to the V.A. Clinic when the weather was bad and there was no way for me to get there. Whenever I was hospitalized he would visit me and would leave me large handfuls of dimes and quarters for use on vending machines and on pay telephones, despite my protests. He insisted on helping me because he believed I had accomplished a lot for workers when I successfully sued the company.

In the evening my brother Bill and his wife Joanne, along with my sister Dorothy, came to visit me.

My brother Bill asked me if I knew what caused my stomach bleeding.

I related to him how my stomach bleeding was caused by the miracle drugs they were giving me for my arthritis. Bill, a very sensitive person, looked sad. To add some levity to the atmosphere I said, "The reason they call those drugs miracle drugs is because it's a miracle if they don't kill you."

But that did not go over very well so, after a moment, I said, "The doctor put me on a blonde diet."

Stephanie, who had been talking to Dorothy said, "No, he didn't. He put you on a bland diet."

"A bland diet!" I said, trying to look surprised.

"Yes, a bland diet."

I then looked back at Bill, clicked my thumb and middle finger, gave a short downward swing with my fist and said, "Dammit, I thought he said blonde diet! Oh, well, missed it by that much." I showed him how much by holding my thumb and index finger about an inch apart.

Bill and Joanne laughed. Then Bill added, "Yeah, you missed it by a hair."

On the fourth day after my surgery I was moved to a private room in an area called "Skid Row" where the more seriously ill patients were kept. It was six o'clock in the morning when I got there.

Since I was not allowed to eat or drink anything, I was getting some nourishment from the I.V., plus getting fluid to keep me hydrated.

But soon after I entered the room my I.V. stopped working. The nurse played with it to try to restart the flow. She adjusted the needle in my vein and injected a small syringeful of saline solution through the needle to try to clear it, but nothing worked.

Finally she took the needle out and said she would try to get hold of a doctor. When she returned she said the doctor was not available.

I looked at her. She was a pretty woman in her early thirties with dark hair and eyes.

"You know how to put in a new I.V., don't you?" I said.

"Yes I do," she said firmly, "but I won't."

I was taken aback by her refusal to do what nurses had been doing on a regular basis.

"Why not?" I asked.

"Because I need the doctor's permission."

"But you already have the doctor's permission," I countered.

"No I don't. You already had the I.V. when you came here."

"I know that," I said with frustration. "That's because the doctor had ordered it."

"Look, I'm very busy and don't want to argue with you. When the doctor becomes available I'll bring it to his attention." Her eyes flashed and she sounded a bit miffed.

"Wait a minute, nurse!" I called out as she was moving to leave.

She stopped and turned to face me. "What is it?" she said, taping her foot impatiently. Suddenly, to me, she looked ugly.

"Let me explain why the I.V. is so important to me. I have kidney stones and a chronic infection, and the doctors told me to drink plenty of water every day. If I don't get my fluid, my kidneys could get into a lot of trouble."

"We all have our problems," she said. "I'll try again to get the doctor." She turned and, in a flash, was gone.

I could not believe what was happening. It would have been so easy for her to put a new I.V. into my vein, I would have been getting my much-needed fluid and my problem would have been eliminated. But, because of her stupidity and lack of compassion, I lay there in the bed with a tube in my nose and hooked up to a wall suction that was pulling acids out of my stomach. I was a virtual prisoner, isolated from everyone except the moronic nurse and left exposed to possible kidney damage.

I could not get my poor kidneys out of my mind and brooded over them.

Anguish and frustration grew close to panic as I realized that the doctor was not coming. I put on my call light and waited for the nurse.

About ten minutes later she came into my room and said, "What is it?"

"Have you been able to get a hold of the doctor?" I asked.

"No he's still not available," she said.

"Then put in the I.V. so I could get the fluids I need."

"I told you before I can't do it without the doctor's permission."

"Goddammit! Don't you have even the slightest inkling of my kidney problems?"

"Well, I've been told nothing about your kidneys," she said, as she took the nearly full urinal out to empty.

When she returned, I pleaded with her to put in the I.V., but it all fell on deaf ears.

As she left, the last thing she said was, "You'll live."

I could hear her fading footsteps moving up the hallway. "Drop dead, you dumb bitch."

Slowly I resigned myself to waiting for the doctor. I had been a patient in this hospital often enough to know that patients seldom win against the system.

It was a terribly frustrating and helpless feeling to be caught once more in the hospital's sinister web, especially when only a short while ago I was heavily involved in running a third-party political campaign in the City of Mullins.

It had been about twelve hours since my I.V. had been removed and I was no longer urinating.

I put my call light on hoping to get some other nurse. After quite a wait, the bitch came in. "What is it?"

We were back on the Merry-Go-Round. "Did you get in touch with the doctor?" I said.

"No, he's still not available," she said, impatiently.

"Are there any other doctors available to put the I.V. in?"

"They're all very busy today," she said.

"What if someone was dying, would a doctor be available?"

"But you are not dying, and I am very, very busy myself," she said as she flaunced out of the room.

I was left with my mouth wide open, just staring at the empty doorway. Why me? I thought. If those sonofabitches had not restarted my bleeding I might have been home by now with my stomach intact, far, far away from this goddamn Alice-in-Wonderland madhouse.

Chapter 7

Finally at 6 P.M., after I had been dehydrating for some twelve hours, a second shift nurse came in. She was cheerful and efficient, and expertly put the I.V. needle into my arm. I was again getting my vital fluids. She was a god-send. I would have been at peace with myself had it not been for my wondering just how much my kidneys had been damaged from the long dehydration.

Later the surgeon, a large, solidly-built man with a substantial waist line and a full black beard that made him resemble a jolly pirate, came in and shut off the suction machine to see if my stomach could tolerate it. It did.

The next morning the surgeon pulled the tube out of my nose, and I had breakfast: apple juice, clear soup, jello and tea. At dinner and supper I had a continuation of the clear liquid diet.

The following day I was put on a heavy liquid diet, and the day after that, on solid foods. Because my stomach was smaller than it used to be, the doctor told me I would have to eat smaller meals, but more frequently.

My hematocrit went up from 28 to 30 and I received two more units of red blood cells to bring it up closer to normal.

The doctor removed the small stitches from my stomach, but left the big ones still in. He also removed the stitches from my right ankle.

The doctors said I was doing good so they removed the I.V. from my arm and, when I got weighed, I was surprised that I was only 121 pounds compared to the 138 pounds before surgery. They were giving me five feedings a day. At mid-afternoons and in the evenings I received snacks from the kitchen, such as a sandwich with chocolate milk, custards or other puddings.

At last, twelve days after surgery, I received two hard-boiled eggs and savored the albumen and other high nourishment that would give me a quicker parole from the hospital.

At noon they needed my private room for a female patient, a former WW-II WAC, so I was transferred to a room with four beds. I liked it better because there were other patients to talk to.

The big jolly bearded surgeon came in with three interns. He had a hearty, laughing disposition and seemed to find the world a hilarious place to live in. I would have bet anything that in the Operating Room he was a cut-up. He showed the other doctors how to remove belly stitches. After making a couple of key snips with his scissors, in one quick swoop, he yanked the big stitches off in one long fish-bone like piece. All I felt was a slight tug. Everyone, including me, laughed, and was amused by his magnificent antics.

A rhuematologist came to see me. We talked about the duodenal ulcer I had. He said that people with Ankylosing Spondylitis were of higher risk for ulcers than the general population, even if they were not on irritating drugs. He mentioned that colitis also fell in that risk category. I was not exactly thrilled with this information, but I felt I could live with it as long as I could stay free and away from the hospital where ulcers were more likely to develop. At last, fifteen days after my stomach surgery, Stephanie and I left the hospital on my discharge.

But as Stephanie and I walked some distance toward the car, my muscles began to ache and I felt as if I weighed a ton. The problem was that I was just not yet acclimated to walking such long distances. Stephanie told me to lean on her. I put my left hand on her right shoulder and, with the support of my cane in my right hand, I walked the rest of the way with reasonable ease.

When I went on my next Renal Clinic appointment, the doctor was surprised when I told him I had part of my stomach removed. The Renal Department was not even notified that I had been in the hospital. "They should have at least let us know," the doctor said, "so that we could've advised them on how to control your kidney problems."

I was also surprised that Renal was not notified. But on second thought, it was not at all that surprising, given the hospital's haphazard communications system.

I described to the doctor how I had been deprived of water for twelve hours and that I believed I had sustained some kidney damage, and that while the hospital was busy working on a patient's primary problem, it was at the same time inadvertently adding on other problems.

The doctor, a tiny cog in a vast machine, just shook his head. Doctors were as helpless as patients when it came to trying to make corrections in a hospital. Yet it seemed to me that too much specialization in medicine had caused the hospital to become fragmented and compartmentalized with each sphere of influence jealously guarded, and the hospital, like a large worm cut into many pieces, moved blindly in every direction at one time while the patients, those helpless and pitiful so-and-so's, were simply trampled on by all this hair-raising chaos.

Therefore, it was virtually impossible for one doctor to treat the whole person. One doctor specialized in ear, nose and throat, another in heart disease, another in liver, another in kidneys, another in hangnails and another in dandruff, on and on. Perhaps, because of the profound complexities of many diseases, specialization may be necessary and the holistic approach impractical, but at least if a centralized communication system could be set up in the hospital that would have kept track of each patient's movements through the various departments and immediately notify the appropriate ones about what was happening to the patient, there might not be so many serious complications and malpractice suits. The computerized communications system could also keep track of patients' X-rays and sound an alarm when high levels of exposure were reached, and it would not be very expensive.

I realize that there is a place for expensive diagnostic machines, but, as long as I am sounding off with righteous indignation, I might just as well mention my belief that doctors are leaning too heavily on these tools and are losing the art of diagnosing.

Anyway, after my stomach surgery, I was afflicted with terrible stomach discomforts after every meal. I would experience a lot of gas, nausea, sneezing, stomach aches, heart palpitations and cold sweats. In the beginning, I assumed that my stomach was not yet healed and that, with the passage of time, I would eventually tolerate food better. But even after some months had passed, I was still unable to eat. The very thought of food made me nauseous. Everything tasted unpalatable and bland, no matter how it was cooked or how many spices and flavors were added. A mere mouthful of food, especially meat, chicken or fish, would bring me to the edge of vomiting. But I tenaciously hung on, swallowing bite after bite, chewing the food to a pulp, forcing myself to finish each modest meal. But invariably, in the middle of every meal, I would suddenly gag and heave up gas in loud, involuntary belches. Where, in the past, I had a voracious appetite and eating had always been a pleasurable experience, my appetite now was non-existent and eating had become a nightmarish ordeal. Every time I sat down at the table it was like being mauled by wild animals three to four times a day just to stay alive. And even after enduring each of these ordeals, I would suffer a couple of more hours of stomach spasms which would force me to take to my bed to get some relief. Therefore, my whole life revolved around the grueling task of eating, then lying helplessly in bed. It was a painful, futile and useless way to live, and the thought of ending it all began to cross my mind frequently. My optimism, by this time, was torn and bleeding and barely breathing. Yet a shred of life still remained in it and I clung to it, trying hard to revive it.

In a mood that was more pessimistic than optimistic, I went with Stephanie for my appointment at Surgical Clinic. There, I was examined by the bearded surgeon, and I told him of the problems I was having. He said my stomach would feel that way for a while, but I should keep eating small meals. That was exactly what the hell I was doing. But, I told myself, perhaps I was being to impatient. Probably, in a little while longer, I would begin to see a silver lining.

Then at the Renal Clinic I received the anti-nausea medication Campazine, which helped a little, and I was able to force a little more food into me. But basically, my problems still continued.

Along with these problems, I also found it more difficult to walk. Prior to my stomach surgery the glue in my left hip prothesis had become loose, making that leg painful and unstable to walk on, but with the aid of a cane I managed to get by. Then, after my stomach surgery, something had happened to my right hip, either in the Operating Room while I was unconscious or during the stretcher-to-bed transfers. Ever since then my right hip prosthesis had also become loose, making it difficult to put my full weight on it. Therefore, since then, I had had to use two canes to help me walk.

Around December, both my knees began getting inflamed and painful, and six Tylenol tablets per day were not helping any. My stomach, as it was, precluded my using any of the more effective drugs such as Indocin and Aspirin, which were anti-coagulants. All I could do was to continue on the Tylenol and hope the inflammation would eventually subside.

Back at the Surgical Clinic, a young, friendly doctor told me there were no traces of blood in my stool. He listened to my stomach with a stethoscope and said it was good with plenty of activity in it, but he did not know why I was still having so many stomach problems.

He suggested I take Gelusil, which might help alleviate some of my nausea. Then, on reviewing my chart, he changed the Gelusil to Basaljel. He said Gelusil, which I had been taking for years because of my arthritis pills, was bad for my kidneys. Basaljel, on the other hand, would not harm them. "Why in hell didn't someone tell me that years ago?" I said. "Doctors had been treating me one piece at a time, giving me medication that helped one part of me while damaging another part of me."

The young doctor, who was writing out the prescription, looked at me, and said, "I know how you feel. I'm sorry that such things sometimes happen."

When I got home and used the Basaljel I found that it did not help my stomach. My stomach and I were one big disaster area. Worse of all, I had not been able to write. Books and stories I had started were gathering dust on my desk. My life was ridiculous, a day-to-day struggle just to exist like a half-alive vegetable. I do not know how often during those months I had seriously thought of packing it in simply by giving up. In my weakened and debilitated state, it would have been the easiest thing in the world to do. The struggle just to exist without really living was just too, too damn much for me.

Yet, despite my burial under tons of pessimism, my stupid optimism, though badly mangled, still somehow kept beating inside me. No matter how impossible and hopeless things looked, it was just not my nature to be a quitter.

I have always been fascinated by how every creature on earth struggled tenaciously for survival. Animals trapped in leg hold traps often chewed their leg off to escape death. Countless other examples of men and other creatures in unbelievable struggles for survival could be listed. Why was that? I had always wondered. Little by little I began to ascertain that it was in every living creatures' genes, genes that have evolved from the very beginning where the strugglers survived while the apathetic drifters perished, on and on, until only the creatures with the struggling genes became dominant.

But why, and for what purpose? To me those questions were still a big mystery, and they were something we can only speculate about. I had speculated on this many times and had come up with some plausible conclusions. One of my favorite ones that I seem most comfortable with was that life had sprung, not only on earth but throughout the entire universe, out of electrical currents that had animated matter and used it for its own purposes. Life had evolved from the very simple one-celled bacteria on to the more complicated multi-celled animals, and then on and on to the more complex forms of life, such as Homo Sapiens, which was still evolving. And if we do not blow ourselves up, we would evolve to the point where our intellect and especially our awareness, which will never be lost—the collective awareness of every creature that had ever lived and those that will live in the entire firmament—will give birth to the most ultimately supreme being in the universe. The same supreme being that poor mankind has been worshipping for such a long, long time, long before the supreme being was even born, and who ultimately will be us.

Okay, so maybe my concept may sound too far out for some people, but when dealing with the unknown, I believe that my speculations, that the struggle for survival has a purpose, are as valid as anyone else's.

Besides all that, there was Stephanie who made it all worth while for me. Without her, I was sure I would have given up the ghost a long time before.

Determined to survive, I went to my next Renal appointment where the doctor checked my ankles, which were swollen, listened to my heart and said it was all right, then felt the heat in my swollen knees and concluded that the swellings were due to arthritis.

At home I found that Basaljel was also contributing to my nausea, so I stopped taking it and satisfied a long-standing urge for chili. I ate a bowlful of it with gusto, making my stomach and me very happy. All this time, since my stomach surgery, I had been avoiding foods that were full of acid and salt, and apparently, with all the antacids I had been taking to try to end my nausea, my stomach had become too alkaline. From then on, I cynically decided to avoid the doctors' conflicting advice and pay more attention to my own body signals so that I could start getting better again.

The January weather was terribly cold, and a big blizzard that had begun the day before was still continuing, so that it made it impossible for me to get to the V.A. for my appointment one day with the Arthritis Clinic. Stephanie stayed home from work, and only emergency vehicles were on the road. My black friend, Jack Fernandez, phoned me to ask if I was able to get to the V.A. I told him there was no way I could walk with my two canes over the snow and ice to my car. He said for me not to worry about it, he would be down in half an hour. When he arrived with his four-wheel-drive vehicle equipped with snow tires and chains, he maneuvered it up close to my front porch. The sky was gray and fine granular snow was still sweeping down in a cold, driving gale. My porch was covered with hard snow and ice, which left Jack undaunted. He carried me piggyback-style over the treacherous ground. After getting me into the car, he drove me through the snow-drifted roads and got me to the hospital, where he waited for me in the lobby.

A few days later I had an appointment with a dietician. I weighed 114 pounds on her scales. She discussed with me a high-calorie diet. I told her it sounded good but my stomach could only tolerate a limited amount of it. She gave me a quart of MCT Oil (Medium Chain Triglycerides) to take as prescribed. The oil was supposed to help me absorb fat.

Although my stomach still gave me trouble and my appetite was still poor, I nevertheless learned to deal with it to some extent and I felt better, at least enough to allow me to get back to my writing.

About six months later, after getting into bed, I felt chilly and could not get warmed up, and I could not sleep. Then, around midnight, despite all the heavy bed covers, I began to shiver uncontrollably. The shivering became very violent, and there was a pain in my left side just below the rib cage. Right after that a heavy throbbing pain suddenly manifested itself in the middle of my back, between the shoulder blades. The pain throbbed sharply with each heartbeat, then penetrated, like a knife, through my back to my breast bone, and I thought I was having a heart attack.

Stephanie became very excited but managed to hold herself together to call an ambulance. Two attendants carried me out on a stretcher and I rode with an oxygen mask in the rickety old ambulance, feeling every jarring bump in the road. Stephanie followed in her car.

In the Emergency Room the EKG proved negative. I had blood and urine tests, X-rays, and then I was sent to the fifth floor with an I.V. line in my arm. In the ward Amphicilin was intrduced into the I.V. to treat another serious E-Coli kidney infection.

The next morning, they brought me down to X-ray in a wheelchair with the I.V. bottle hanging on a short pole in back of the chair, and left me waiting in the cold hallway. There were many patients ahead of me and I asked a passing technician what part of me they were going to X-ray. She answered, "Chest and belly." I pointed out to her that I had already had them done yesterday. The young woman checked the records and found that I was right. She said the order she had was the same one used yesterday, therefore I did not need to be X-rayed. I was pleased that I had questioned it, at the same time I was angry that a patient had to question every damn move made by hospital staff members. Consequently after a long wait for an escort, I was finally wheeled back to my room. Being sick and weak as I was, this hassle was hardly helping me any. My kidneys had stopped working when I arrived in the ward, I was unable to urinate. My tissues, especially my legs, were swollen with fluids and toxins, and I was feeling utterly miserable.

The following day I was sent to Ultrasonics to have my kidneys, pancreas gland and gall bladder checked. The tests lasted for quite a while and, after getting out of there, I finally began passing urine, and I began feeling a little better. The tests did not reveal anything unusual. In the ward, I was given a cup of purple, bitter-tasting Potassium to drink.

From then on, I began to improve, except for the deep

nausea which prevented me from eating anything. The doctor said it was due to the slight increase in my kidney function, but thought it would clear up.

Gradually, the puffiness from fluid retention and the severe nausea began to subside. The doctor said I was doing well, and my B.U.N. (Blood Uric Nitrogen) was now down to 95 from 110.

Later, my B.U.N. went down to 70, but my ankles were still swollen. The doctor explained that because of my poor appetite, especially in protein intake, my albumin was very low. This caused the fluids to leak through the vein walls and become absorbed into the tissues.

An Immunologist came to examine me, then he said they would put me on a drug that would keep my urine sterile to prevent further attacks of blood poisoning. Further attacks, such as I had, could prove fatal. I never saw the Immunologist nor his mysterious drugs again.

A couple of days later, I went to X-ray for an I.V.P., but after a couple of exposures, the doctor cancelled the test because the kidneys did not absorb the dye.

The next day, I had my gall bladder X-rayed, but there too the dye did not absorb well, so that also was cancelled.

The following morning I was again in X-ray, and again the gall bladder did not absorb the dye. The X-ray technicians wanted to give me a dye to drink, then I would have to wait until 12:30 to get X-rayed. I balked at that idea, explaining to them that I did not want to go without water till then, and why (if I did not worry about my kidneys, no one else would). They then came up with another concoction, whereby I would only have a half-hour wait. I agreed, and drank what tasted like egg nog. A half hour later, I was X-rayed.

Stephanie arrived early Saturday morning with my clothes so I could go home on a weekend pass. But they told us we would have to wait until my new doctor came in to see me.

My new doctor was a woman, Dr. S. was her name. She told me the gall gladder X-rays were still not clear enough. After returning Sunday evening from my weekend pass, I received Citric of Magnesia. Then in the morning, I went to X-ray for an I.V.P. But because of schedule problems, it was again cancelled. I then got a small snack of a breakfast.

Later I was sent to Nuclear Medicine where I received an injection in my vein for a liver scan. Dr. S. told me last Friday's gall bladder X-rays did show stones. Good grief, I thought, don't I have enough problems? I didn't need lousy gall bladder stones, too.

At 11 A.M., I was in Building #2 getting dye put in my veins in the "drip" method. The kidneys absorbed the dye so slowly that it was 2 P.M. before the entire series was completed, and I also missed my dinner. Rather than wait for an escort to take me back, I walked to Building #1. Because I was debilitated and weak from hunger, I barely made it back. Dr. S. told me to drink plenty of water to wash out the dye from my kidneys. She also said the previous day's liver scan showed that the liver was normal. I was grateful to hear good news for a change. At 4 P.M., I was sent back to Building #2 for one more follow-up X-ray.

One morning, while eating breakfast, without any warning whatsoever, a young man wearing a cowboy hat came in and asked me if I was ready to leave for a kidney scan X-ray. The nurse said I had to leave immediately. I left half of my breakfast, got into the wheelchair and was brought outside to a van which had a wheelchair lift. Before I realized it we were headed for the major local hospital.

At the hospital, they gave me 12 ounces of bitter, clear fluid to drink. Then a doctor injected more dye into my veins. I soon became nauseous and threw up. The attendant told me this sometimes happened with this dye. They then got me on the table, which moved me into a circular, tunnel-like contraption. When the X-rays were taken, the young cowboy shipped me back to the V.A.

On Friday, as I was getting ready to leave on a weekend pass, Dr. S. told me the kidney X-ray scan did not come out clearly. I was very worried at constantly being overexposed to unnecessary X-rays, including the many that never developed properly, but I was still aware that nobody could beat the system. We hear that the U.S. delivers the best medical care in the world. I say bullshit!

Later, Dr. S. prescribed Darvon for me instead of Tylenol, which she said could cause kidney damage. Now they tell me. First I was told to take my arthritis medication with meals only after my stomach lining was eroded, then I was put on Basaljel instead of Gelusil only after the Gelusil had damaged my kidneys, and now I was put on Darvon because Tylenol, that I had been taking for years, could damage my kidneys. How in hell could a patient possibly win?

Anyway, the Darvon seemed to work better on my arthritis than Tylenol did, but Darvon tended to make me drowsy and sluggish.

I had a consultation with an orthopedic surgeon, and hoped to hear him say that a hip replacement would be as easy as replacing a car hubcap. But instead, he explained that they would have to chip out all the old glue, which was a very tedious and difficult task, and that the glue was harder than my bones. It was a bigger operation than the original one was, and there was the danger that my femur could split apart. Also, because of my renal problems, they did not think I could tolerate such a long operation very well. And my bones had become thinner from my renal problems. I would be better off walking with my two canes. If it should reach the point where it became too painful to walk, then it might be worth the risk. Well, that information took the rest of the wind out of my sails.

Again I was sent to Building #2 with no breakfast or water. This time it was for I.V.C. X-rays of the gall bladder. Despite the dye, the gall bladder did not become visible until one and a half hours later. They finally got all the X-rays completed at 1 P.M., after which I had my dinner, which was cold and too unpalatable for my stomach.

Later Dr. S. told me the X-rays showed no stones in the gall bladder. The other day I was told the X-rays did show stones. But as long as I had a choice, I decided to accept the last X-rays as valid. After all, I would prefer my X-rays to show no stones.

After I inquired, Dr. S. told me my kidneys were functioning at only a fifty percent level. It was not happy news, but I felt that fifty percent was still better than no kidneys and was adequate enough to keep me going for the rest of my life if I could only stay out of the goddamned hospital.

At last I was discharged, broken down a few more notches, but at least I was still alive and kicking.

On Saturday evening, Stephanie and I were on our way from Mullins to Trumbull to visit my brother Joe. As I was driving the car I found myself missing turns at cross roads as though I were a new driver. My mind and my reactions were very sluggish. My eyes were going out of focus whenever I shifted them from one object to another, and despite the activity of driving my car, I felt drowsy and the realization that I was spaced out, from all the Darvon I was taking, frightened me. We were on the Merritt Parkway, where I found it difficult to keep the car from drifting over the white line in the road, and in all the years that I had been driving, that was the first time I felt really frightened and unsure of myself. I was not even sure I could pull the car over to the soft shoulder in a safe manner to let Stephanie drive. Therefore, I asked Stephanie to let me know whenever the car started drifting to either side of the road, and I continued onward at a slower speed till we reached our destination. Needless to say, when we left my brother's house, Stephanie drove us both home.

I continued taking my Darvon regularly. It gave me a warm glow of numbness that helped relieve my arthritic pains, but, while I was on them, I stopped driving the car.

Some time later, I went to the Arthritis Clinic with badly swollen and painful knees and elbows. I was not only finding it almost impossible to walk with my two canes, but I was also feeling depressed, knowing the doctors no longer had any miracle drugs that I could safely take. All the doctors at the clinic were strangers to me. Two of them examined me, but did not know what to do for me. They called in their superior, who pondered over my medical records, then prescribed for me seven milligrams of Prednisone daily. I felt better emotionally because I was getting some help.

The Prednisone, I found, reduced the pain and inflammation considerably. But I only had enough for one week, and there was a "No Refill" sticker on the bottle. I assumed that this medication could only be taken safely for short periods at a time.

As the days passed, my arthritic pains gradually returned. Then, over the next few weeks, my ankles all the way to my knees became severely swollen with adema. These swellings were unusual and I suspected that they were caused by something other than arthritis. Later the swellings subsided, but they still remained in the ankles. Also my appetite, as bad as it was, began growing even worse so that I could barely finish half a modest meal. And this was happening even though I was no longer on antibiotics. My weight was down to 114 pounds, which included all the excess fluid I had on board.

At the clinic, I was given excellent advice on how to gain weight. I was given a case of "Ensure," which was a chocolate-like drink with 250 calories in each of the eight-ounce tins. The only trouble was, nobody was able to tell me how I was supposed to get all these wonderful calories and vitamins into my belly. Every tin I tried to drink, no matter how slowly, only brought me untold hours of agony and stomach distress, so that, after getting down only a few tins of the stuff over many days, I gave it up completely.

In September of 1978, in addition to the badly swollen ankles, I discoverd that my left leg was also swollen all the way up to just above the knee. At the back of my left knee I felt a hard lump that was giving me some discomfort. Then a very sore spot appeared in my left calf muscle and, when I tried to walk, I found it increasingly difficult to put my full weight on that leg.

Then, in the evening, it was so painful to step on, that I had Stephanie drive me to the V.A. Emergency Room. The interns diagnosed it as plebitis. Because it was a Saturday there was only one radiologist on duty and he was at the major local hospital working on another emergency. We waited from 9:30 P.M. till 1:40 A.M. before the doctor arrived. In the X-ray room, he did a Venegram and confirmed that there was a vein blockage which was therefore thought to be plebitis, though it was not plebitis. As soon as the diagnosis was completed, the doctor and the X-ray technicians vanished like bandits, leaving Stephanie and me out in the deserted hallway. There were no signs of life anywhere, except for the biggest cockroach we had ever seen in our lives. Without exaggerating, I would say it was around two inches long and built like a Mack truck! It was walking at a leisurely pace past the stretcher I was reclining on. Stephanie quickly pushed my stretcher to the elevators, but we did not know where we were supposed to go from there. Just as we were making the decision to go back to the Emergency Room, a security guard came along and we told him about our dilemma. He called someone on his small radio and soon a nurse arrived and brought me to 5E, to a private room. By now it was 2:30 A.M., Sunday morning, at which time Stephanie left for home.

An intern interviewed me and I was attached to a machine that controlled the blood-thinner, Heperin, which was running into my I.V. Being in a supine position all this while was very uncomfortable for me, and the I.V. in my arm, plus my aching back, limited my movements. My left knee ached me so badly that I requested a pain-killer and a sleeping pill. But the pain continued and would not allow sleep to come. A heating pad wrapped around a wet towel helped only slightly, but because the knee was kept rigid by the wet pack it only caused the pain to become excruciating. I called the nurse to have it removed, but I was told I had to have it on because this was part of the treatment for plebitis. (It was taken off periodically to allow me to bend my knee to get some relief.) During what was left of the night, I only slept for brief periods, and even then they were restless semi-sleeps.

It was not till Monday night that I was finally allowed to sleep without the hot pack on my left leg and I slept a lot better.

Besides the so-called plebitis on my calf, I also had a large, tender swelling on my left hip, which I had first discovered on Sunday evening when it was only the size of a marble. By Tuesday it had grown to the size of a golf ball. But none of the doctors who were treating me were able to diagnose it. They sent me to have my knees and hips X-rayed to see if there might possibly be an infection in my artificial hip joint. Scenes of devastation twirled through my cranium. I visualized myself being wheeled into the O.R. and having the entire hip joint removed, leaving a void that would perhaps make me unable to walk forever. The anguish and worry continued to torment me till I was told the X-rays proved negative. There was no infection in my hip joint, and this news brought me great relief. Yet there was still this mysterious swelling in my hip which I could feel growing larger almost by the hour.

In the afternoon Dr. C., from Arthritis, came in and examined my leg carefully. Then, to the other doctors who surrounded my bed, Dr. C. pointed out a number of telltale signs that indicated the vein blockage in my calf was caused by a ruptured Baker's cyst. Once the other doctors were put on the right track they all agreed that it was indeed a Baker's cyst and not plebitis. The dummies had been giving me the wrong treatment, a treatment that could have easily caused me to bleed to death.

I was taken off the Heperin and was given vitamin K into my I.V. to help build up my blood-clotting factors. The large lump on my hip was finally diagnosed as a hematoma which was caused by internal bleeding. Because my crit had dropped from 28 to 24, I was given two units of blood, the blood that I would not have needed had I not been on the unnecessary Heperin. If it had not been for Dr. C., who seemed to be the only doctor in the hospital who knew how to diagnose, I was sure I would have definitely bled to death.

On Wednesday, I had both my swollen knees drained and steroids injected. Then I was sent to Ultrasonics for an echo study of my calf.

Since my stomach problems continued dominating my life, I related my problem to every doctor who treated me. This time, after investigating post-stomach surgeries, they came up with some answers. First of all, since the size of my stomach had been drastically reduced, it was no longer able to hold food to partially digest it before slowly releasing it into the small intestines. What it now did was simply dump it in wholesale lots directly into the intestines. Since the intestines were unable to handle such large volumes of undigested food, hence came the stomach pains, heart palpitations, etc. This they called the "Dumping Syndrome." To correct the problem, they came up with a high-protein and low-carbohydrate diet with no sugar or fluids during meals. For breakfast I received four slices of bacon, two eggs, and a slice of toast with margarine and no tea or coffee or fruit juices. At mid-morning, I got cottage cheese and crackers. The rest of my meals were also high protein and low carbohydrates. My stomach began feeling so good that I began smiling again, thanking the doctors for coming up with the solution to my stomach problems. (Little did I know at that time what this high-protein diet was doing to my poor kidneys.)

Anyway, as the days passed, I was told the lab had found TB germs in my urine. (Just what I needed.) But a couple of days later they told me further tests were negative. They said the first test may have been a contaminant that had gotten into the test in the lab where there are many such germs. What good was a contaminated lab where life-and-death decisions are often made?

I was sent on a stretcher to the orthopedic doctor's office where he examined my hip and the X-rays. He believed the lump on my hip was a ruptured muscle. This, of course, confirmed the cause of the hematoma, which had stopped growing since I had been off Heperin.

On the seventh day, I was sent to Therapy for some mild exercises. I now weighed 105 pounds and looked like a cadaver.

On the eighth day I started walking a little. In the evening I received a liquid diet in preparation for an upper and lower G.I. series. There had been some traces of blood in my stools, and although the bleeding had stopped since I had been on the high-protein diet, they thought it would be a good idea to get my stomach and intestines checked anyway.

On the following morning, after getting enemas, I was in X-ray. There I received a barium enema and I was fluoroscoped and X-rayed. Then, in another X-ray room, I had four more exposures made to see how much of the barium still remained. I returned to my room at 10:30 and was given a light breakfast. Then they gave me a bottle of Citrate of Magnesia to drink in order to clean out the remaining barium, which was an unhappy ordeal for my stomach. But before I could finish it, I was hustled into a wheelchair and brought to Building #2 to have my lungs checked. I had to blow into a tube on a machine that registered my lung capacity and strength. When that was done, I decided not to sit there waiting for an escort and instead walked back to Building #1. (A patient may sit in his room for days without a single test, then suddenly be inundated by them.)

I was extremely thirsty when I got back to my room and I immediately finished the Citrate of Magnesia. Just then my dinner tray arrived. Because I had drunk the Citrate too fast I was bloated, but I finished most of my dinner anyway. Immediately after that I was again hustled down to X-ray. But when I got there, I learned that the doctor who did the barium X-rays was now at the major local hospital, so I was brought back to my room. At 2:30 P.M. I was again brought down there. The doctor told me the barium did not go all the way through to the other end of the colon because he had stopped it when he thought he had reached the other end. He said it was his fault, but from what he did see of my colon there did not seem to be anything there of significance. I was scheduled for another test next Friday.

When I got back to my room the doctor told me I would have to get another lower G.I. series completed before they could start on the upper. It was an incredible torment to have to go through and I contemplated telling them to go to hell with their goddamned tests.

The next morning, my doctor told me my kidney function was low and my B.U.N. was 120. He asked me if I were drinking enough liquids. I told him, no, because I had to fast for the G.I. series and the enemas had drained out considerable fluids, followed by so many other hassles that I just did not have enough time to drink much water—which I had to do slowly. Also, I was passing far more urine than normal, which was leaving me quite dehydrated. In the evening, I had an I.V. put in my arm to ensure that I got enough fluids.

The next morning I received another Citrate of Magnesia to drink. When I had finished half of it my doctor came in and told me not to drink any more of it. He told me the test would have to be postponed because my B.U.N. was still 110. They might try to do the test the next day.

As I lay there in bed thinking about it, I finally decided I would refuse tomorrow's test. I got out of bed and, pushing my I.V. pole, I walked to the doctor's office and told him about my decision. To my surprise, he told me they had also reached the same conclusion. They thought that the elevated B.U.N. was caused by my prolonged dehydration. It should return to normal in a couple of days, after I had sufficient fluids. (Hell, I could have told them that in the first place, and I now regret that I did not have sense enough to intervene sooner. Instead, like most patients, I had the tendency of going along with everything the learned doctors told me.) My creatine was still all right, he added, which made me grateful for at least that much.

The next morning I had no breakfast and was sent to Ultrasonics, where I had my pancreas checked. This test at least did not require all the elaborate pre-test preparations such as long fasts and enemas. Besides, I was now getting my fluids through the I.V. In the echo room I was hungry, thirsty and cold. (This room and all the other X-ray rooms were always like huge walk-in refrigerators where, in the thin johnny-coat, you could expect to shiver like a jackhammer, and possibly die of pneumonia.) I got back to my room at 11 o'clock and drank a large cup of water and ate a cold breakfast.

In the afternoon I learned that my B.U.N. was down to 90. I was told that, while I was in Echo, four renal doctors came and had a consultation with my doctors. They too had reached the same conclusion that my elevated B.U.N. was due to dehydration.

Tuesday morning I received no breakfast. I informed the nurse, who checked the kitchen and found that they had made a mistake, thinking I was scheduled for another X-ray. An hour later, a small unappetizing breakfast that was quickly thrown together was brought to me. Yes indeed, a hospital is no place for sick people.

At 5 P.M., when I was finally discharged, Stephanie and I left the hospital posthaste. Everytime I was hospitalized my kidneys sustained some degree of damage, and I had also developed a chronic cough, either from the dirty air conditioners in the summer or the warm air ducts in the winter, and it would take almost two weeks to recover from it at home.

I think that if the ASPCA ever learned what patients went through in hospitals they would take them out and send them to dog pounds where they could be given some degree of humane treatment.

Chapter 8

Around the beginning of October 1978 I was feeling very cold no matter how much warm clothing I was wearing. And in bed, despite the heaviest bed covers, I would shiver uncontrollably. I would even add a heating pad, which radiated a lot of heat before my shivering would subside. My temperature was running around 99 to 100 degrees, and despite the fact that I had these symptoms before and they were caused by a urinary infection, I convinced myself that it was only a slight virus infection or a malfunction in my metabolism. I kept lying to myself that it was probably nothing serious and would eventually pass, and I continued deceiving myself, determined to weather this storm at home simply because I dreaded like hell having to go back to the hospital.

But by the third week, the chills got worse, and I was feeling weak and lethargic and completely out of sorts. Stephanie told me I looked awful and I should not wait any longer and she convinced me to go to the Emergency Room. It was 4 P.M. when we got there.

A doctor examined me and we waited in the room for hours, then I had my chest X-rayed and I was brought to the Medical Intensive Care Unit. There they made a small incision and inserted a catheter into my neck vein to run it close to my heart to more accurately monitor my blood pressure. It

took two painful tries before they finally got it in the right place.
Because my blood had lost its clotting ability, the incision continued bleeding. They put a stitch in it, but it still continued oozing blood. Finally, the next morning they took the catheter out completely and stitched up the incision.
I asked a lot of questions and was told my kidneys were not working and my B.U.N. was 250, an unbelievably high reading. My pancreas was inflamed and not working right. My electrolites were way out of the ball park, and I had a serious case of acidosis. With all those out-of-wack readings, it was a mystery that I could remain alive, let alone walk into the Emergency Room, a nurse told me.
They took me on a stretcher to Echo and X-ray. Judy S., a lovely, dark-haired young student doctor who was assigned to my case, went with me. Through the entire ordeal she had been a great comfort to me listening to my complaints and answering my many questions about my condition.
My pancreas gland was inflamed, so I was not allowed any food. Also I was told that I needed dialysis immediately. I was stunned by this news. I knew I had kidney stones and occasional infections, but it just never occurred to me that I would ever need dialysis. It was so shocking to me that I just could not believe that it was happening to me. They told me that kidney failure and Pancreasitis were both treated by a thirty-six-hour peritoneal dialysis.
I signed a consent form and, while I was still in bed, one of the doctors, under sterile conditions, made a small incision just under the belly button, and pushed in a plastic tube which popped through the skin to a depth just between the skin and the intestines. Then the tube was surrounded by a bandage, a long tube was attached to it and two quarts of glucose fluid, hanging from a pole at the bedside, were slowly drained into my peritoneal cavity, uncomfortably

filling it up and causing me to hurt like a pregnant woman—I think. When the two quarts of water were all in, they let it sit in my belly for twenty minutes before they let it drain out. As soon as the peritoneal cavity was empty, they again let two more quarts slowly fill it. The first drainage that came out was red with blood. But the nurse assured me that the bleeding was due to the incision and would soon clear up. But each drainage continued to come out dark pink and it continued during the entire thirty-six hours, so that I had to get blood transfusions along the way.

After the dialysis was completed, they pulled the tube from my stomach, stitched the incision, then bandaged it. My B.U.N. was down to 80, and my kidneys began to slowly recover, but I was still not allowed to eat anything because of my inflamed pancreas. I later learned that my acidosis was attributable to the high-protein diet I was put on; my weak kidneys could not handle the overload.

Although I was getting some nourishment through my I.V., I did not receive anything to eat or drink for seven full days. Around the fifth or sixth day my mind began to be plagued by thoughts of dying from starvation. I remembered reading somewhere that when people were starving for an extended period, and when they were finally given food, their stomach could not accept food and they died anyway. "Could this be what would happen to me?" I asked myself. It frightened the hell out of me. I asked the nurse about it, and she said she did not think so. But I could tell by the way she said it that she was not certain about it. Everyone who came to my bed was asked this question, but none gave me a convincing answer. Even Judy S. did not really know the answer to my question, but she promised me she would investigate it and come back with the answer.

After a while Judy came back smiling and told me that, under controlled conditions, prolonged starvation was generally no problem. What they did when feeding resumed was to start a patient on a clear liquid diet, then heavy liquid until the stomach got acclimated to solid food again. Although I was still gravely ill and in critical condition, I was quite relieved by her answers. She, like my wife Stephanie, had a heart of gold and they both helped to keep my spirits high.

My blood pressure was 200/110 and I was getting a large assortment of drugs to try to correct my body chemistry.

One of the many drugs I was being given had caused me to hallucinate. I was in a weird land, a land filled with grotesque and illogical happenings. It first manifested itself on my mind when Stephanie was visiting me. She was standing at my bed, leaning on the side rails talking to me. As she talked, I watched her face turn dark yellow, then rapidly dark brown right before my eyes, and suddenly her words were incomprehensible to me and she looked, not only like a total stranger to me, but like some threatening extraterrestial being. A chill of fright ran through my spine, and I said, "What happened to your face and hands?" She looked at her hands with surprise, and said, "Nothing happened to them, why?" As she said this her face and hands suddenly resumed their natural color. I described to her what I had seen. She thought that perhaps it was the way the light reflected through the window on her green dress. But whenever I watched her face for more than two or three minutes, her face would again begin to turn yellow and I would have to divert my eyes to get rid of the yellow tinge.

The next morning I found it difficult to deal with my surroundings. To me, everything appeared alien and familiar at once. Time and space seemed to overlap and run into each other like crazy, hazy illusions. For example, when I tried to reach my hand to the side railing, in order to roll over on my side, I grasped a handful of air instead of the railing.

The railing was not where I had seen it. But by reaching out for what seemed like a very, very long distance, I finally was able to reach it.

Later on as I was lying on my back, I languidly put my hand on my chest (I was wearing no pajama tops), then suddenly it occurred to me that the buttons and wires that were monitoring my heart were missing. There had been a half dozen of these buttons glued to my chest, and I found there was not a single one left. Because of my stiff neck, I could not look down, and frantically ran my hand in circles over my entire chest, searching for those elusive buttons which just simply no longer existed. This strange occurrence frightened me and brought me close to panic, not because the buttons were missing, but because I could not fathom how anyone could have removed them without my knowledge. Determined to get to the bottom of this mystery, I resumed sweeping my hand over my chest, going higher and higher toward my neck. But there did not seem to be any end to my chest, it just continued on and on for what seemed like several feet. At last my hand did touch the buttons, all of them were there and accounted for, and I realized that what I had originally thought was my chest was actually my belly.

On my wrist was a black-and-blue spot that was caused by an I.V. infiltration. As I gazed at this spot, it slowly turned pitch black. I called the nurse and showed her my hand. She said that there was nothing wrong with it, that it was not black as I was claiming. Surprised by her attitude, I looked at the hand and indeed it was back to normal.

When the nurse left, I again looked at my hand. To my astonishment, my hand again went into its color change routine. I again called the nurse and again the hand returned to normal. It was playing tricks on me, I thought. I could see it as plain as day, but as soon as someone else came to look at it, it resumed its normal color.

Later on, I saw the heavy green curtain drawn on one side of my bed so that I could no longer look out at the activity in the unit. I asked the nurse to draw the curtain back. She said that the curtain was already back. I told her that it was not back all the way. She handled the curtain and showed me that it was all the way back and could go no further. I frowned and realized that the curtain was indeed all the way back.

I was not sure whether I had fallen asleep after that or not, but the next thing I remember, I was lackadaisically lying on my side watching the nurses moving about the unit. I did not know how it happened but my bed was now completely reversed. My head was where my feet had been and my feet were where my head had been. Yet it did not in the least concern me, I just kept watching the activity of the unit. Suddenly I noticed that the curtain was again drawn, but not completely because I was still able to see the entire unit. At this point I had to use the urinal which was hanging on the side of my bed way out of my reach. I called for a nurse and was surprised that none of them had responded. In Intensive Care, the nurses always respond to a patient's needs. Now they were moving about completely oblivious to my calls. This time I shouted loudly for a nurse, but they continued to ignore me. Some even passed close to my bed without any sign that they heard me. I became almost hysterical and I shouted and shouted at the top of my lungs. There they were still going about their business without hearing me at all. I paused to ponder the situation. I reasoned that either the nurses had suddenly all become stone deaf, or my voice was not getting to them. I knew that sound traveled through the air and I knew that I had been making sounds, very loud sounds which I was able to hear clearly. Then a frightening chill ran through me. I must be in a coma, I thought. I was comatose, a vegetable—no, not a vegetable yet, because my mind was still working. But my mind was trapped in a non-functioning body. It was locked tightly, perhaps sealed forever inside my cranium, with no way out and no way to ever again communicate with the outside world. I was banished from the world of the living and confined to a world of total isolation. Yet I was clearly able to hear and see the outside world, but it was like watching a movie on a deserted island where no living thing existed. As frightened as I was, I tenciously resolved to remain calm.

When a nurse came to my bed to take my blood pressure and pulse, I asked her if she had heard my yelling. She said she did not hear any sound from me. I then realized that the bed was again back in its original position with the head of the bed being where it was in the first place. Comprehending that I was carrying on a conversation with a nurse, I began to wonder whether she was actually real or whether I was just imagining her. Unable to distinguish between real and unreal, I said, "Are you real?" "Of course I'm real. Here, touch my hand," she said, as she extended it to me. I took hold of her hand and smiled with relief. She was indeed real and I was indeed in touch with reality.

She told me that a drug they had been putting in my I.V. to try to correct my heart skips had caused me to hallucinate. She said that while most people were not affected by it, a few were, and apparently I was one of them. I asked her if it would affect my mind forever. She said no, it would pass when the drug wore off.

I was gratified to have learned this, and although the hallucinations continued throughout the rest of the day, they no longer frightened me.

These illusions came over me in periodic waves and I would see strange things that were not there, and I would casually observe them and wonder about them and even begin to wonder whether the real world was actually real or whether we were in a mass hypnotic state, just imagining it all.

In late afternoon I was transferred from Intensive Care to the ward and placed in a private room. My friend from the plant where I worked, Jack Fernandez, came to visit me as he had been doing right along (he was an outpatient in the Alcoholic Ward). He noticed that I had no wristwatch so he gave me his very expensive watch and told me to keep it. I did not want to take it, but I told him I would borrow it for a few days.

Jack was on his way out when Stephanie arrived. They happily greeted each other, then he left. He was a true friend and Stephanie and I liked him very much.

While Stephanie was visiting, I felt the shimmering waves of another round of hallucinations coming over me. I saw a strange animal, something like a mole, walking on the wall close to the ceiling. Despite my knowledge that it was only an illusion, the animal seemed so vivid and real that I was certain Stephanie would also be able to see it. "Look over there," I said, pointing to the wall. She told me she saw nothing. I glanced at her, then back at the animal, which was suddenly no longer there. Frightened by my behavior, she went out to get the nurse. Then the nurse brought in an intern who examined me and asked me a few questions such as: "What is your name? Do you know where you are?" Of course I knew my name and where I was, because by then the delirium had passed.

That night I found it impossible to fall asleep. I spent most of the night reading a book. Then around 1:30 A.M., I felt a burning sensation in my esophagus and it gradually developed into a severe heartburn. I asked the nurse for some antacid. No matter how much I argued, she refused to give it to me because it had not been ordered for me by a doctor. Later the heartburn became so severe that it caused me severe chest pains. When I called her again and told her about my chest pains, she called the intern. Two interns arrived and checked my heart with an E.K.G. which did not show anything abnormal. But to be on the safe side, they shipped me to the Coronary Intensive Care Unit where I spent the rest of the night under observation lying on a hard stretcher because they had run out of beds. In the morning I heard a woman's voice calling my name, "Michael! Michael!" over and over, and someone was shaking my shoulder vigorously. I sluggishly opened my eyes and saw Judy S. with a very worried expression on her face. When I said, "What happened?" she let out an audible sigh and said, "Thank God you're awake! I had been trying to wake you for some time. You were in a coma!"

Puzzled by this, I asked her, "Why, what happened to me?"

"Your tissues are overloaded with fluids. People in that condition could go to sleep and never wake up again. We're going to have to increase your diuretics to get rid of the excess fluids."

Blood tests revealed that I had no heart problems and I was taken back to the ward, this time in a room with four beds. They said my chest pains were probably due to heartburn. All that pain and aggravation was caused by a stupid nurse who had refused to give me some antacids.

It appeared that I had been soaking up the fluids from the I.V. bottles and I was not passing much urine. The increase in my diuretics increasd the urine flow and the I.V. flow was slowed down to a minimum, but most of the excess fluids still remained and I was drowsy and spent most of the days sleeping soundly. When someone tried to wake me up it required a lot of effort. I had been on a liquid diet since leaving Intensive Care and my blood pressure, despite all the fluids I had on board, was down to 98/72.

I had been receiving large quantities of sodium bicarbonate every day on a regular basis to help neutralize some of the toxins in my system.

Jack Fernandez dropped in and gave me a brand-new Timex wristwatch he had just purchased. I did not want to accept it, but he insisted that I take it, saying it was a Christmas present. I relented, feeling very touched by his generosity. There are many more goodhearted people in the world than anyone can imagine.

My somnolent days continued. I spent most of my days and all of my nights sleeping deeply. And even when Stephanie came each evening to visit me, I would sometimes inadvertently doze off. Dr. Judy S. told me that, although I was getting rid of some of the fluids, there were a lot left that the kidneys were still unable to handle. Stephanie had brought a copy of my novel *We Ain't Going Back No More, No How* for Judy, who loved literature, and she and I had long discussions about it. She was very pleased to receive it. She also said that I might have to get one more thirty-six-hour dialysis run before I got discharged. I kept my fingers crossed hoping I would not need it.

Feeling terrible, I was sent in a wheelchair to Occupational Therapy on the seventh floor. There they measured the range of motion in my arms and the strength in my hands, which were not what they used to be. I was given a few simple arm and hand exercises to do for half an hour.

In the afternoon I got a touch of the chills. My hematocrit had dropped for some unknown reason. They took blood to check for infection. Later they found that the low crit was due to a lab error. (So what else was new!)

All week I had had diarrhea, which was draining what little strength I had left. Doctors thought it was caused by Queenadin, which they were giving me for my heart skips. A couple of days after stopping Queenadin, my diarrhea ended, and most of my excess fluids were gone. They also told me that the nausea I had been having was due to my kidneys not functioning properly. They had been taking vials of blood from me every day and my hematocrit had really dropped. I was given two units of blood. As bright as doctors are, they sometimes come down with spells of stupidity.

No breakfast or fluids were given to me in the morning. I had to wait till noon before Ultrasonics finally called for me. But none of the tests came out because I was constipated and full of gas. This long fasting had again caused me to become dehydrated and my B.U.N. went up to 130.

When I got back to my room I felt weak and tired, and I sat on my bed for a few minutes to rest. A ninety-year-old man in the bed across from mine asked me if I needed help to lie down. I realized that I was in far worse shape than I had suspected.

I did not get a weekend pass because I still had the I.V. in my arm hydrating me. Three renal doctors came to see me. They told me my creatine was up to eight. If the hydration did not bring it down, then dialysis would be considered.

Luckily for me the hydration helped my kidneys and my blood values moved closer to normal. Although I was quite debilitated, I nevertheless was feeling better and more alert, and then I was discharged.

At home, life for me had become even more arduous than it had been. I was no longer taking Prednisone for my arthritis, not since my pancreasitis attack which the doctors suspected was caused by Prednisone, and my joints were stiff and painful. At the Arthritis Clinic I had my right knee drained and injected with steroids. This treatment, which caused long-range damage to the knees, helped, but it was only a month or so before I again needed more steroids.

At one of my Renal Clinic appointments, I told the doctors about my weakness and my painful arthritis. He sympathized, then read off the numbers from my last blood test. My hematocrit was down to 20, creatine was 6.5, B.U.N. was 120, but everything else was normal, and my urine infection was gone. My kidneys were still functioning, but not well, and he explained the advantages and disadvantages of the two types of dialysis, hemodialysis and peritoneal dialysis. Although I saw the handwriting on the wall I was still not prepared to accept dialysis. I thought that if I took good care of my kidneys, they might possibly improve their acuity to better filter the blood, and I might not need dialysis for many years to come.

January 1979, at 1 P.M., Stephanie got me to the Arthritis Clinic. I did not have an appointment till the next week, but my knees were so painful that I just could not wait any longer. Little did I know what it would be like to go there without an appointment. First I had to wait till my chart was brought up from subground. Then we were sent to Evaluation, which was at the other end of the building. After a waiting period, we were sent to the lobby, where we waited for a very long time before my name was called. Then I was sent to the Emergency Room, where I had to take off all my clothes, and a doctor examined me. I told him I only came in for a steroid injection for my knees, but they insisted that this evaluation was necessary when a person came in without an appointment. Suppose I had come there to deliver a telegram!

There were no traces of blood in my stool, but they found that my blood count was only 17. It was 20 a week before. Although I was concerned about the low reading, I knew that when my arthritis flared up I usually became anemic. The examining doctor got so alarmed by my low crit plus my weakness that he strongly urged me to get admitted. I refused, but when another doctor agreed with the first one, I reluctantly went along, and at 6 P.M. I was in 5W.

The next day, Dr. C. came to see me. He said they might

put me on Motrin for my general arthritis, plus steroid injections in my knees. A hematologist suggested a bone marrow test to pinpoint the exact cause of my anemia. Later, another doctor told me a bone marrow test might not be necessary. They were able to get adequate studies from my blood tests. After dinner he drew fluid from my knees, then injected steroids. Later, an I.V. was put in my arm and I received a blood transfusion.

The following morning my joints felt better and I felt stronger. My hematocrit was now 25. The doctor ended his tour and was replaced by another doctor who told me that hematology still wanted a bone marrow test. He said, after the test, I would be able to go home. Anxious to get home, I decided to get it over with. It was a knee-jerk reaction that I later regretted.

The doctor had me lie on my stomach with a pillow under my chest so that my face was off the mattress. From the back of my pelvic area he aspirated the bone marrow and also got a bone biopsy. It hurt, but not quite as much as in 1969 when I had the first one done.

In the afternoon, a nurse who taught dialysis came to talk to me. She said that both hemo and peritoneal would work well for me and I would be able to do it at home. At the sound of the word "home" my ears perked up. Peritoneal was easier for one person to handle. The permanent tube implanted in the stomach cavity must be kept sterile at all times to avoid peritonitis infection. If infection did occur, it could be treated in the hospital with a seventy-two-hour flushing with antibiotics plus a few days of antibiotics taken orally. I was pleased to hear how easy it would be. (Little did I know.)

At 6 P.M. I was discharged from the hospital.

But two days later, on Sunday, February 4, 1979, Stephanie again drove me to the Emergency Room. My right hip was locked in agonizing spasms. The muscles in front of my thigh up to the groin hurt very badly when I tried to straighten my leg. The pain was excruciating whether I stood up, sat down or lay down. It became unbearable, and Stephanie drove me to the hospital and brought me to the Emergency Room in a wheelchair. I was helped onto the stretcher and the nurse did the usual tests while we waited for the doctor to arrive. When he finally came in he asked a large number of questions, but he did not know what to do. After a couple of hours of agony I was finally given an injection of morphine. It dulled my senses and reduced some of the pain, then I was sent to have my hip X-rayed. After that I was returned to the Emergency Room, where I lay on the examining table in terrible agony, and the doctor did not know what to do and left the room for a very long time. Then more doctors arrived and I was finally taken to 5W. I was pretty well doped up by then, having received three more morphine injections.

The next day many doctors came to examine me, including Dr. C. Dr. C. was the one who thought my pain was caused by a hematoma in the back of the hip, probably from the bone marrow test. It turned out to be exactly that.

The doctor who did the bone marrow test put an I.V. in my arm, then I had a number of blood tests. My right hip and groin were still painful when I tried to straighten my leg. Later I got two units of blood.

On the third day I was bloated from all the narcotics I had been getting, and I was again overloaded with excess fluids. At night I could not sleep because I found it very difficult to breath. I slept in a chair all night, which helped me breathe a little easier, but my breathing was still labored. The doctor gave me an injection of Lasix to help me pass some of the fluids that were overloading my tissues and lungs.

Later he discovered a rubbing sound in my heart beat. A fluid buildup around my heart had caused the heart to become constricted, which was why my breathing was so labored. I was given oxygen and a few other doctors listened to the heart rub. Then I was taken to the fourth floor where my heart was scanned by echo. The doctor thought I should be on dialysis as soon as possible. The way I felt, very sick and miserable, I was definitely going down for the last time, so dialysis no longer posed any great fear for me. Instead, I now began to view it as a lifesaving raft.

As I lay in bed with my head raised to help me breathe, I ruminated over my dilemma. If I did not come to the clinic to get my knees injected and if I had not accepted the bone marrow test which told them nothing more then they had already known, I would not have received the hemotoma and then the morphine, which caused me to become bloated with fluid that restricted my heart so that now only dialysis might possibly save my life. I closed my eyes and clenched my teeth in frustrating tightness. Stupid! I was goddamm stupid! stupid! stupid! for allowing the simple-minded doctors to do this to me! Now, heroically, they were trying to save my life! Surveying my limited resources, I concluded that there was still enough of me left not only to recover but also to function adequately for perhaps a very long time to come, even on dialysis. Because of all the writing I still had ahead of me, I had no doubt that I would make it.

The dialysis surgeon came to tell me he would operate on me immediately (it was February 9, 1979). He asked me for Stephanie's phone number and said he would call her to let her know.

After getting a couple of quick enemas, the stretcher arrived. Just after that, Jack Fernandez, with a big smile on his face, came in to visit me. When he found I was going to the O.R., his black face became solemn. He walked along with me while I was being wheeled toward the elevators. At the elevators, Stephanie came out from one of them. She was out of breath, having just run here all the way from the north parking lot. I told her it would be a simple operation. She went with me to the third floor, then as I was going into the Operating Room, she went to the Waiting Room.

In the Operating Room I was covered all over with green sterile sheets, had an I.V. put into my arm and blood pressure taken. Then the surgeon swabbed my belly with Bethedine. Then he injected lydicain into the site just below the belly button. After that he made a small incision and put in a tube to run some water into my stomach cavity to form a "lake." Then he worked the permanent catheter into place. Except for the occasional pressure discomforts, there was almost no pain at all. I was in there for an hour and a half, then I was taken to the Recovery Room and Stephanie came in. I smiled and told her that everything went well.

From there I was brought to M.I.C.U. and was soon being dialyzed. I still needed the oxygen to help me breathe. A number of heart doctors came in to check my heart. Then I was taken to a room where the doctors inserted a catheter into my neck vein and into my heart and injected a dye and looked at the fluoroscope and took some X-rays.

Later they told me that the sac around my heart was loaded with water which was putting enormous pressures on the heart. To correct that would require cutting away the sac. That, of course, would mean major heart surgery. Without the operation, the pressures could cause the heart to stop beating. The only trouble was, my chemistry numbers were so far out of normal that the operation would become highly risky. They said I had about a fifty-fifty chance. Without it, my chances were nil. Aware of my very debilitated condition, I felt certain that I could not survive surgery. In surgery, even with a fifty-fifty chance, I would not have the control I felt I needed to survive. Whereas without the surgery, even with my chances being nil, I would at least be sort of in command of my own destiny. Like my Timex watch, I knew my heart could take a lickin' and still keep on tickin', and that was the course I intended to take.

To my surprise, the surgeons told me they would hold off on the operation in order to give dialysis a chance. Perhaps the fluid around my heart might dissipate. That was all I needed. With the help of dialysis, I now had a fighting chance.

On the following day I was still being dialyzed, and beginning to feel better. My breathing was no longer a problem, so I happily dispensed with the oxygen. Even before the surgeons later confirmed it, I knew the fluids around my heart had dissipated. Stephanie said she had a feeling that I would make it, just from what she had seen in my eyes.

I was dialyzed for two and a half days. My B.U.N. was down to 73. In the afternoon I was transferred back to the ward. I went back to M.I.C.U. for one more eight-hour dialysis. After that I went three times a week, 12 hours a day, to Building #2 where I was dialyzed on the automatic peritoneal machine. The machine worked well, giving me very little discomfort compared to the more crude method used in M.I.C.U.

On Friday I requested a weekend pass and the doctor granted it. But Stephanie phoned to say her car had broken down and had to be towed to a garage. The temperatures outside were sub-zero. On Saturday the car was repaired and she drove me home for the weekend. Although I was feeling a lot better, I was quite a bit below par.

On Monday, at 7 A.M., I was taken to Building #2 for my dialysis. At noon the machine had broken down so I was taken off. (Each time I was put on and taken off the machine it was done under sterile conditions. The nurse wore a gown, rubber gloves and a mask. And I also wore a mask. Then the nurse removed the bandage, cleaned the area around the catheter with Bethedine, then to it attached a sterile tube that led to the machine. It ran approximately two quarts of dialysate fluid into my stomach, shut off automatically for twenty minutes, then started up again to drain out the fluid. When the fluid was completely out of my belly, the machine continued the cycle all over again. It was far more complicated than I had thought, and my stiff neck made it impossible for me to see my belly to be able to do this sterile procedure alone.)

I was again short of breath and felt very weak, so the doctor checked my heart with an E.K.G. and took blood samples. My crit was still 25. I was sent back to my ward in Building #1, then I had a chest X-ray. A doctor told me that, because my kidneys no longer produced a certain hormone, the bone marrow no longer made red blood cells as fast as it used to.

On Tuesday I was again being dialyzed in Building #2. I felt much weaker and my breathing was getting more difficult. The doctor checked me over and sent me to Echo on the fourth floor of Building #1. They found fluid again around my heart, so they sent me back to M.I.C.U. Then I was taken to the fluoroscope room where doctors put a catheter in the vein in the right side of my neck and ran it to the heart to monitor the pressure. Then they stuck another catheter into a vein in my right groin all the way to the heart. Then I was sent back to M.I.C.U. and put on dialysis and given oxygen to breathe. I had absolutely no appetite and I was able to eat very little when my trays arrived.

The dialysis continued for about two weeks. Doctors said I was finally improving. My crit was 37. The doctor removed the catheter from my neck vein, then I was able to get up to sit in a chair for a while.

When dialysis was stopped, I was transferred back to my ward. In the evening I again developed shortness of breath.

The next morning another doctor checked my heart with an E.K.G., then sent me to X-ray. He said X-rays showed less fluid around the heart than the previous day. He thought my shortness of breath might be due to irritation of the heart from the irregular heart beats. He would prescribe medication.

The next day I was back in M.I.C.U. getting dialyzed and being given Queenadin for my irregular heart beats. For two days I continued getting dialyzed. On the following day I was taken to Building #2 for dialysis.

Jackie, the Renal Dietician, told me I had a very serious malnutrition problem. She insisted that I had to eat more, especially proteins. I described to her how impossible it was for me to eat, and that meat in particular made me gag. I was much worse off than I had been when I first had my stomach surgery. At that time I was able to at least force the food down. But now I could only force down certain foods like carbohydrates, but in limited amounts. Meat was virtually impossible to get down except for a few bites. I was very much aware of how serious my nutritional problem was, and I had been struggling with it ever since my kidneys had failed. I knew full well that if I did not start eating again, the consequences would surely be fatal. But as incredible as it may seem, even with all my efforts and all my determination, I could not overcome my stomach's violent reaction to food. Although institutionalized food may be light years away from being considered fit for human consumption, it nevertheless was at least edible. But to me everything, especially meat, tasted putrid.

I had my chest X-rayed, and a doctor told me the fluid in my lungs had decreased and my heart looked good. That was the first time I had heard of water in my lungs. But this good news brought little joy to me. I was now confronted with a problem that overwhelmed everything else, leaving me totally helpless and unable to fight back. Even Jackie had reached the end of her rope in trying to get me to eat. She therefore, after exhausting all her efforts, told me the only other course they had left was tube feeding. At this point I was willing to try anything.

A doctor inserted a tube into my nose down to my stomach. Later, on an I.V. pole, they hung a bottle containing Isocal, which was a complete liquid diet, and a machine, controlling the flow, allowed so many drops per minute into my stomach every day for twenty-four hours a day. I was supposed to get a certain amount of this fluid every day. If it dripped too fast my stomach got bloated. If it dripped too slowly I did not get my full quota. Often the tube would clog up and the nutrition would stop flowing, sometimes for hours. When it was restarted again some of the nurses, to make up for lost time, sometimes rushed the fluid into my stomach, which caused me terrible discomfort. After I complained about it, this practice was stopped, and my quota simply fell behind. In the meantime, I was still getting my three meals a day and ate very little of them.

In March, arthritis doctors drew fluid from my right knee and injected steroids, and a young woman therapist came to my room every other day to help me do some simple leg exercises in bed. I did practically no walking all this time.

As the weeks dragged on, even with the tube feeding. I still felt weak and lethargic, and there was no sign that I was improving. In fact, in every way, my chances were looking hopeless and very bleak. I was inexorably sliding down the slippery chute of doom, and there was absolutely nothing I could grip onto to stop this precipitous downward slide.

Chapter 9

The head nurse in the dialysis unit had a private discussion with Stephanie and asked her if she would be willing to take two weeks off from work to learn how to operate the machine in hopes of dialyzing me at home. Stephanie, who had observed the temperamentality of the machine and the frequent shrill warning sounds each time there was a malfunction, plus the very delicate and highly sterile procedure for putting me on and taking me off, did not think she could handle such a heavy responsibility. Because she had to work every day, she felt that she would be too tired to do the dialysis properly, and she would never forgive herself if anything went wrong.

The nurse later told me that, because of my arthritis, I would not be able to handle the machine alone. Then she told me that Stephanie had rejected the two-week training. I was disappointed at first, but as I thought about it, I realized that it would definitely be too much of a burden to add to her already overburdened schedule.

My dialysis doctor told me that peritoneal dialysis was not working well for me, as it did for most patients, plus it was taking precious protein from my body. Hemodialysis, he said, would give me a more complete dialysis and it would only require six hours, three times a week, instead of the twelve hours that peritoneal took.

A month later I was transferred to Building #2, in a ward

close to the dialysis unit. At 3 P.M. I was sent to Physical Therapy till 4 P.M. every other day to do simple arm and leg exercises.

Because most dialysis patients no longer urinate, potassium builds up in their bodies and can interfere with the heart beat. If potassium levels reach a critical point, the heart can stop altogether causing heart failure. My potassium was very high. The doctor took five vials of blood, then injected something intravenously. Later he took another blood sample to try to determine why my potassium was climbing.

By this time, with problems piling on top of problems, I had become so thoroughly depressed that I just lay on my bed in woebegone placidity and had very little interest in what was happening to me. I did not exactly give up all hope, it was just that the whole thing had become too, too much for me, so I withdrew as a participant and left everything up to the doctors and to nature. I had simply worn out my will to fight back and was unable to get my second wind.

Jackie told me that they would continue the tube feeding and stop my trays for a few days, till they could unravel the high-potassium mystery.

Six days later I was again getting my food trays. This time I was able to eat a little more, but not enough. I was also getting the Isocal.

Finally the doctors discovered that it was the Isocal that was causing my high potassium, so my Isocal intake was reduced.

A day later the dialysis surgeon inspected the veins in my arms and I signed a consent form for him to operate on my left arm to create a fistula (dilated veins) to give the dialysis needles easy access to the veins.

Later, a psychologist came to talk to me. He was very young and he wanted to know why I refused to eat. I resented his attitude right from the beginning and I told him that I did not refuse to eat, I was just unable to eat. I mean, the way he came on, it was as if he thought I was a malingerer or was just being obstinate or something. No matter how much I kept explaining to him why I could not eat, he kept insisting that I had to eat, that I had to force myself to eat no matter what. I said to myself, here was a guy who was young and healthy telling me, who had been through the mill and has had half a stomach removed and renal failure, that I should force myself to eat. I did not need his advice to tell me what I had to do. What I needed more than anything in the world was for someone to tell me how in the hell I could actually get the food into my belly. Luckily, his first visit was brief.

The next day I was given no breakfast and nothing to drink. A nurse scrubbed my entire left arm with Bethadine. I had a chest X-ray and no dinner. Then at 1 P.M., on a stretcher, I was taken to Building #1 to the Operating Room. On the operating table I was covered with green sheets and had an I.V. put into my right arm, and my left arm was extended out. The surgeon washed it down with Bethadine and injected Lydicaine. Then he made an incision close to the inside of my elbow. Then, after probing for a vein and an artery, he and another doctor stitched them together. After that he stitched the incision, bandaged it, and the operation, which took two hours, was completed. Back in my room a sling was attached to my wrist and tied to an I.V. pole to keep my arm up in the air to prevent it from becoming swollen.

On Saturday I went home on a weekend pass. On the Monday, after I got back, the surgeon removed the stitches from my arm.

Rheumatologists had concluded that, instead of continuing injecting my swollen knees, it would be better to get my knees radiated. But the Radiologist refused to do it, not only because of the possible cancer risks, but because he did not think it would do any good.

In the evening, the psychologist came to my room to talk to both Stephanie and me. He first began by talking about my inability to eat, then when he learned that I had no will to do anything but sit and brood over my many misfortunes, he badgered and admonished me with very rational arguments. Despite the sense his arguments made, they did nothing to stir the sluggish mud in my veins. It was evident that something vital had broken down in me. Not only did I find it difficult to smile anymore, but I had also lost the ability to laugh at things I once considered funny. I was no longer my old self anymore. I just could not look forward to very many tomorrows. Yet I could still remember how, a short time ago, I had a firm handle on myself. I had long ago surmised that the awesome universe contained all the knowledge that existed, and so I had plugged my mediocre mind into it and inhaled hungrily from its vast creative outpourings. But now, because of events beyond my control, I had become unplugged from this energizing cosmos, and was left drifting aimlessly through a silent void. And here was this young psychologist telling me what I already knew, that I should pull myself together—in effect, that I should plug myself back into the stream of life. Sure, that was easy for him to say. But what he did not understand was I was not in this dilemma because I had failed to perceive the enormity of my problem. It was just that, when my body had broken down beyond a certain point, my endurance ran out, and it no longer mattered what I thought or did, it was ALL SENSELESS. For me everything was all over, kaput, ended. If Stephanie, whom I loved very much, could not put my shattered psyche together, then how on earth could this still-wet-behind-the-ears psychologist possibly help me?

Nevertheless, the psychologist was very persistent and finally persuaded me to accept an assignment, which was to write something for him to read the next time he saw me.

That evening I wrote about the dangers of nuclear power. The next day he came to see me in dialysis and read my article. He liked the article very much, which surprised me because I had somehow perceived him as a straight-laced, establishment person—which he probably was—but he told me he was also an environmentalist. Consequently, we talked for a considerable length of time about our wasteful economy built on obsolescence, so forth and so on. This sparked my spirits back to life a little and I realized that I was beginning to care about things again. Yet my eating problem still existed. I was still forcing food into my stomach but getting down not nearly enough to make up for my deficit.

Jackie told me that dialysis patients' appetites are sometimes helped by zinc tablets. The doctor had ordered them, but, for some reason, the V.A. Pharmacy was unable to get them. After three weeks the zinc tablets did come through and were given to me three times a day. Gradually my appetite increased till eventually, for the first time in almost two years, I actually began feeling some hunger pangs, but my stomach capacity was still limited. Still, even though I could no longer gain weight, I could at least hold my own nutritionally.

I continued my twelve-hour, three times a week runs on peritoneal dialysis, and the doctors said that I was making some progress. I would be feeling better when I finally got on hemodialysis, which would remove all the toxins from my blood stream. I was very sick all through that whole period and was looking forward to getting on hemodialysis.

At last my incision healed and I had a fair-sized fistula sticking up on my arm. I went for my first hemodialysis treatment.

I chose a recliner chair instead of a bed. My fistula was not yet fully developed and the nurse had difficulty trying to get the needle into the vein's center. The punctures felt like small drops of molten metal landing on my skin. By the time both needles were properly set, my arm had enough tracks for me to be in danger of arrest by a narc agent. It took two horrendous hours before I was finally on the machine. I watched my blood run up the clear plastic tube through an artificial kidney, then down into a drip chamber, then back into my blood stream in a continuous flow that was supposed to last six hours.

But three hours later the alarm sounded, the machine shut down, and two nurses found that one of my needles had clogged up. One of the nurses removed the clogged needle and then tried to put another needle into another vein to try to get the blood from the machine back into my veins. But by then the blood had clotted in the machine and I lost several cc's of blood from my already anemic body. It was a terrible experience. My arm was swollen with hematomas and my back ached from the awkward chair. It was not a full dialysis, but it was enough for the first time. I was told that the first few times were the hardest, but once the veins in my arm became larger and tougher, then everything would go much easier.

I got back to my room and took a nap, and then when Stephanie came, we left on my weekend pass.

At home Stephanie helped me climb the back porch steps, and though I enjoyed being home I felt too weak to do much of anything. My new novel, which was only half completed and which I had left untouched for six months, was still on my desk. I tried working on it, but I had neither the energy nor the proper mental clarity to accomplish anything, and the little that I did manage to write I later threw away.

On Monday, at 7:30 A.M., I was back in hemodialysis. This time I chose a bed instead of the chair and it took only three tries before the needles were put in my veins. Because of all the blood I had lost in my first hemodialysis my crit was down to 16, which did not surprise me and which accounted for my extreme weekend weakness. The doctor told me that they would give me a blood transfusion. When they tried to crosstype my blood, the lab found antibodies in it, so they delayed the transfusion till the next day. (I had a low-grade fever at this time.)

After giving me two units of blood, the doctor said I might get discharged the following week. After five months of being hospitalized I was glad to hear this, yet I felt terrible and knew I was still too sick to go home. Perhaps by the following week I might be feeling a lot better.

Gradually the veins in my arm expanded to the point where there was less trouble inserting the needles and I was able to get a few full six-hour runs. In the meantime, I still had the peritoneal tube in my belly as a back-up in case problems developed in my arm. In fact, my arm did become so swollen that I had to go back on peritoneal dialysis for one more run to give my arm a chance to recuperate. After that, as the veins grew tougher, the post-dialysis swellings were less frequent.

Things were stabilizing themselves and I began feeling better and was now eager to go home.

Dr. C. came to my room to see me. He reiterated that radiation was the only thing they had left for me. He did not believe that radiation to the knees would pose any long-term dangers because the knees do not contain any bone marrow. He would try to convince the reluctant radiologist.

The doctors were ready to discharge me, but the radiologist agreed to radiate my knees. When I got to subground in Building #1, the radiologist explained that radiation might be risky. Patients who had their spines and chests radiated showed a significant rise in Leukemia several years later. He admitted that there were no statistics on knee radiation, because this procedure was seldom done. But he believed there were some risks, and the decision was up to me. If I agreed to have the treatment I would have to sign a consent form indicating that I was aware of the risks. I was taken aback. Should I just let my knees go as they were and eventually become a cripple? Or should I risk Leukemia in the hopes that my knees would get better? It was quite a quandary I was in. I decided to take the risk and sign the consent form. I got my first treatment immediately. It consisted of one and a half minutes of radiation for each knee. There were to be six treatments all together—Tuesdays, Thursdays and Saturdays—which would be between my dialysis days and which would spread out to two full weeks.

On Mondays, Wednesdays and Fridays, I was still being brought to dialysis in a wheelchair. There I was weighed, then I lay on the bed and was put on the machine by a nurse without any problems. After I got off, the head nurse changed the bandage on my stomach where I still had the peritoneal tube. (The doctors said the tube would be removed when they were assured that my hemodialysis was consistently running smoothly.) Although my dialysis was running fairly well, there were still occasional swellings of my arm which required hot packs after some of the runs.

A young blonde woman, a lovely and bright person, was my primary nurse at that time. Each nurse was assigned to keep track of the progress of a certain number of patients. Once a month my nurse read me the chemistry numbers that came back from the lab on my blood tests, and there was constant improvement in every one of them.

I was eating better and Jackie had solved my protein shortages by ordering cottage cheese for my dinner tray instead of the meat which I still was unable to eat.

Thursday morning, after getting my knee radiation, I was on a stretcher heading for the Operating Room where the surgeon would remove the catheter from my belly. One nurse put in the I.V. and the other assisted the two doctors. After sterilizing the area on my belly, the surgeon numbed it with novocain, snipped off the catheter at the skin line, then made an incision on the right side at the other end of the tube where he removed the bulb end which had become ingrained inside the tissue. After sewing up the incision he made another one a few inches to the left of my belly to remove the other bulb from the peritoneal cavity. With the tube now out and the second incision stitched, he bandaged it and I was taken to the recovery room where I waited till two nurses from my ward came to take me back.

Saturday, June 9, 1979 was my discharge day. I went to have my knees radiated for my last treatment. My knees were feeling better and were considerably less swollen. When I got back, Stephanie had all my things packed. My physical condition was even poorer than it had been and the knowledge that I would have to be dependent on a kidney machine for the rest of my life was something I had already come to terms with. The main thing was that I was still alive and I was still able to do so many of the things I wanted to do.

Frank, the runner, took me down to the lobby in a wheelchair, then Stephanie drove me home.

At home I was kept busy on my novel while Stephanie worked, and in the evenings we would both relax. I continued going three times a week to the hospital for my hemodialysis treatments. Arrangements had been made by the hospital's social worker for the Red Cross to drive me there three mornings a week and for Stephanie to pick me up after she got out of work at 3:30 P.M.

On one particular day my arthritis was giving me a lot of pain. My elbows and shoulders were swollen and inflamed. The left arm, which was immobilized by the needles, became even more painful till it became unbearable. The nurse put a heating pad under my shoulder and I got some relief.

When the doctor came, I told him about my painful joints. He said he would talk to the rheumatologist about it. My knees, on the other hand, were no longer swollen since they had been radiated.

The surgeon dropped in, took my belly stitches out, then replaced the bandages with two band-aids.

After getting off the machine, my arthritis was so bad that I had to be taken by wheelchair down to the lobby.

After Stephanie drove me home, I could not climb the back porch steps because, since being discharged from the hospital, I could not lift my legs up high enough to reach the top of each step. Therefore she had to lift my leg up on each step so that I could, with the help of my canes, get myself up.

My arthritis was growing more troublesome, so that I needed, besides the heating pad, Tylenol and Codeine to get me through the six-hour dialysis runs.

On Tuesday, after making an appointment, Stephanie drove me to the Arthritis Clinic. The doctor examined my joints. The left shoulder was especially severely swollen with fluids. Dr. C. and another doctor came in to examine me. One of the doctors injected Lydicaine into my left shoulder, then with a syringe and a large needle drew out some fluid. After that he injected steroids.

I continued exercising my legs and one day I surprised Stephanie and myself by climbing the back porch steps on my own. From then on, I no longer needed assistance, at least for a while.

My vision has always been 20/20 all my life, but on September 10, 1979 my eyesight had suddenly become blurred. I found it impossible to read the newspapers.

The next day in dialysis a doctor examined my eyes with his small flashlight but could not detect anything wrong. He made an appointment for me to see an ophthamologist. I got off dialysis an hour earlier and Frank pushed me in a wheelchair to Building #1 on the fourth floor. The Eye Clinic was crowded so I had a nurse call Stephanie to let her know where I would be when she came to pick me up. When the doctor finally examined my eyes, he told me I was nearsighted and also that I was beginning to get cataracts. He did not know how long it would take before the cataracts became "ripe" for surgery, because it varied with each individual. But he did prescribe eyeglasses for my nearsightedness. I later found I was still unable to read!

A few weeks later, Frank pushed me to the Eye Clinic. They could not find my chart, so in between her other duties, the receptionist made numerous phone calls trying to track it down. Finally, after a long wait, they found it, but by then it was too late in the day, so I received another appointment.

I have seen hell raised by patients who had traveled long distances to keep their appointments only to be told to return on other days. Clinics in general are quite chaotic, but the Eye Clinic is the most crowded, disorganized and insensitive one in the whole hospital, where even the most patient of patients lose their patience.

On Thursday the doctor checked my eyes again and found that there had been a change in my eyesight, so a different prescription was written. It was a very frustrating experience. All I wanted was a pair of eyeglasses so that I could begin reading again. Reading had been a very important part of my life and despite all my efforts, plus going to private opticians to try to expedite the matter, six weeks had passed and I was still in limbo.

When I finally got my second pair of eyeglasses, they also were a big disappointment. They never focussed properly and I was able to read just one word at a time. While on dialysis, I found it impossible to read. At home I read with a magnifying glass. Later I went to an outside eye doctor who only confirmed that I was getting cataracts.

On Monday I went to the Orthopedic Clinic to have my right hip prothesis looked at. The doctor sent me to X-ray in the morning, and after a long hassle I was back in Orthopedics in the afternoon. The doctor looked at the X-rays and said there was not much change. He admitted that it was possible that the awkward stress on it could split my femur bone. He suggested that I get it checked every six months. That hip joint, which had been put in at an angle, had been and continued to be a great source of worry to me.

When my primary nurse was transferred to the Home Unit, I was assigned to another primary nurse, a young Italian girl who was very meticulous and good humored, who was like a protective mother hen to her patients. My dialysis had been running smoothly but mostly the same sites were being used over and over again. She told me it would be better to develop different sites to give those most frequently used a chance to rest. She got the arterial and the venous needles in a new site with one try and they worked well.

In the meantime, every single morning I was getting out of bed enduring terrible arthritic pains. Every movement I made was excruciating, which forced me to move at a snail's pace when dressing myself. But the most painful periods were on my dialysis days when I had to rise at 5:30 A.M. and move at a faster pace to get ready for the Red Cross driver to pick me up at 7. After I went to the bathroom and washed up, Stephanie would help dress me to speed up the process. But the pain I had to endure was sheer hell. When the driver arrived, I needed help getting my legs into the car. And this agonizing experience was going on and on without letup. It was bad enough to have to depend on a machine to stay alive, but to have to go through all this never-ending pain on top of it was just too much for me to bear. It was hardly worth staying alive under these conditions. The only way I could see of getting out of this quandary was to simply put a halt to my dialysis treatments. From what I had heard and read, it was one of the most peaceful ways of packing it in. Without dialysis treatments, the urea and other toxins would build up in the bloodstream causing lethargy, drowsiness, a short coma and then the end.

In a last desperate effort, I made an appointment with the Arthritis Clinic. After dialysis, I was pushed there in a wheelchair and was told my chart should be there. I later learned that my chart was not there. Being delirious and helpless with pain, I could no longer cope with these mix-ups. After waiting for an hour and a half, I was finally called into the examining room. By this time Stephanie had arrived from work, so she went in with me. Dr. M., a young black woman, had only a thin folder from Dialysis Unit but not my complete chart. I had to give her the details verbally, but without the chart she was cautious about prescribing anything for me. She called in her attendant, who also examined my left shoulder and elbows. Finally, four thick volumes of charts arrived. All the information about me was contained in them. But not knowing whether my left shoulder was arthritis, bursitis or bone collapse, they suggested I get an X-ray first before they could make a definitive determination on the treatment required. All my hopes for immediate relief collapsed around me. In the meantime, they recommended an increase in my Tylenol and Darvon dosage, which did little good. Stephanie wheeled me down for my X-ray, then we went home.

The head of the Dialysis Unit urged flu shots for all dialysis patients. I chose to have one because dialysis patients were more susceptible to disease than the general population.

The following Tuesday I was back at the Arthritis Clinic. The X-rays showed that it was arthritis in my left shoulder, not bone collapse. Dr. M. and another doctor said that Prednisone in small amounts would be my best medication, but they wanted to wait another week to see how steroids in the left shoulder would work. She injected the left shoulder and I left.

A week later I was back. I told Dr. M. that my left shoulder and elbows had improved but the rest of my joints were still very painful. She took off my stockings and felt my ankles, which were very hot with inflammation. Prednisone and Motrin were the only two medications she could prescribe for me, but each had their own side-effects. Prednisone decalcified the bones and retained fluids in the tissues. Motrin interferred with the platelets making bleeding hard to stop. She decided to talk to the head dialysis doctor to find out if Motrin would interfere with my dialysis.

On Friday she told me she had written a prescription for Motrin. On Tuesday, after dialysis, I got the Motrin, which I took at home with my supper. The next day much of the pain was gone.

Because I needed more support for my legs I had requested a pair of Canadian crutches to replace my canes. After dialysis I was brought up to the sixth floor, where the therapist read my chart, and I explained to him why I needed them. He said it would take two weeks before they came in. Since Canadian crutches were so frequently used by so many patients, I could not understand why they did not have them in stock. I reconciled myself to the two-week wait, hoping my hip joints would hold up till then.

In the meantime, the Motrin I had been taking was becoming less and less effective and my arthritis came back with a vengeance. It was now worse than before I had taken Motrin. When I got off dialysis, I was so stiff I was barely able to walk with my two canes to the elevators.

At home I had been having diarrhea for the past five days, then I became so weak Stephanie had to help me walk. In the morning, to help me down the back porch steps, she supported me on one side while the Red Cross driver supported me on the other side—and she went to work late. At the hospital the driver offered to get me a wheelchair, which I refused, and I struggled to the Dialysis Unit on my own, at a slow pace. I felt that if I started depending on a wheelchair I would never again walk.

The dialysis doctor thought the Motrin might be responsible for my diarrhea and prescribed Lomotil to control the diarrhea.

On Tuesday morning, November 29, 1979, Stephanie and the Red Cross driver again helped me down the porch steps. My arthritis was too painful for me to walk, so when I got to the hospital the driver pushed me in a wheelchair to the unit. The head nurse put me on a machine in a separate room in isolation because my liver enzymes were abnormal. After dialysis, the doctor decided to admit me to the hospital. (It was just as well because I was too weak and in too much pain to try to make it home again.) I was sent to Building #1, 5W. The doctor concluded that my hepatitis was caused by Motrin which I might be allergic to. In the hospital, all I got for my pain was Codeine, and I had to endure terrible days and nights. In the meantime, a lot of blood tests were taken and my liver enzymes were slowly returning to normal. Later, I learned from the nurse that, when my liver enzymes had climbed way beyond normal, the doctor told her that I would be dead before the end of the week. But instead of dying, as the doctor had predicted, I pulled a fast one on him and lived.

Seven days later, I finally received steroid injections in my right knee and left shoulder. During this time, my potassium had risen above normal and my heart beat became very slow and irregular. In the evening they brought me to the Coronary Intensive Care Unit and hooked me up to a heart monitor, and gave me a potassium-absorbing substance to drink and also three enemas to help eliminate some of the potassium.

After breakfast, a technician brought in the dialysis machine and one of the dialysis nurses put me on.

A few hours later my potassium reading came down and my heart beat went back to normal. In the afternoon I was moved back to the ward. A couple of days later my left knee ached, so they gave me another steroid injection. The next day my knee felt better.

Finally, on December 13, 1979, after surviving a near fatal hepatitis attack, I was discharged.

During my next dialysis, a rheumatologist took some fluid from both my knees, then injected steroids into each. He wanted to try injections one more time before sending me back to radiation. When I got off the machine my legs were still very painful. It was not till the next day that I began to get relief.

At last, on January 5, 1980, the Canadian crutches, which were supposed to take two weeks to arrive, finally arrived—after two months. My primary nurse had them for me when I got there in the morning. I found them supremely more supportive than the two canes, and what can euphemistically be called walking was greatly improved.

My arthritis continued its flare-up, especially in my left shoulder. Also I had developed very painful spasms in my lower back. At the slightest sudden movement, the pain would shoot through me like bolts of lightning.

In the morning I again needed help from Stephanie and the driver to get me down the back porch steps. At the hospital, the driver got me to the Dialysis Unit in a wheelchair. A rheumatologist looked at my severely swollen left shoulder, but did not want to aspirate it while I was on dialysis, so he made an appointment for me to meet him in the Emergency Room on the following morning.

In the Emergency Room, the doctor removed several vials of fluid from my left shoulder. Because it was cloudy, he sent the fluid to the lab to see if it was infected. He therefore did not inject any steroids into my shoulder because if it was infected the steroids would only stimulate the germ growth. But he did inject steroids into my left elbow.

The next day I felt well enough to walk to the Dialysis Unit unaided.

On Tuesday, after dialysis, I went to the Arthritis Clinic where Dr. M. and Dr. C. aspirated some more fluid from my shoulder, then injected 1 cc of steroids into it. (The lab had found no infection.)

My shoulder and elbows were a lot better for a while, but on February 26, I was back in the Arthritis Clinic because my arthritis was acting up again. Dr. M. called in Dr. C. who came in with three other doctors. He suggested that I get my knees radiated again, but to hold me over they injected the knees with steroids.

A couple of weeks later my arthritis was back as severe as ever. On Tuesday, March 18, 1980, I again needed help getting down the back porch steps. Practically every joint in my body was painfully inflamed. By the time the nurse had taken me off dialysis, the doctor had already made arrangements for me to be admitted to T4E Ward in Building #2. I had a 103-degree fever.

To bring my fever down and to give me some relief from the pain, the nurses gave me four Tylenol tablets every four hours. At night I sweated profusely. It was no picnic being back in the hospital.

The following day I was brought to Radiation, where I had my left shoulder and both knees radiated. Then I had a chest X-ray. In the afternoon I had steroids injected into my left shoulder and elbow.

On the following morning at 7 A.M. I was brought to the unit in a wheelchair for my dialysis treatment, then I had another chest X-ray.

On Friday I began to feel more limber, but still had a lot of pain. After I returned from my second radiation treatment for my shoulders and knees, the doctor told me the lab had found bacteria in the fluid from my shoulder and gave me two doses of Dankamyicin intravenously. He also aspirated some more fluid from each knee.

The next day, after my dialysis treatment, I was again given a dose of Dankamyicin.

Every other day I alternated between dialysis and radiation, but except for my left shoulder and elbow, the rest of my joints were still very painful.

One day while I was on dialysis, a doctor from the Arthritis Clinic came to see how I was doing. All my joints were very sick and very painful and I told him the radiation was not giving me any relief. He said it might take some time before I felt the effects. Then he admitted that it was possible that it might not work on me the way it did the first time. I then confronted him with the only question I had left: "If the radiation did not work for me, what else is left?" He looked at me solemnly, shrugged his shoulders slightly, then said, "Nothing." Here, after years of struggling with Ankylosing Spondylitis, I lay helpless and at the end of my rope, and a doctor, who specialized in rheumatology, tells me that his bag of tricks is now empty and there is nothing more they could do for me. Suddenly my racing mind spun out of control and skided headlong toward the reaper's sickle, and my emotions ruptured loose a dam of tears that poured down my contorted face. I had wept before over the loss of loved ones, etc., but never over my own approaching demise. The doctor seemed taken aback, and consolingly told me they would have a consultation and try to come up with some solution.

On the following afternoon, Dr. C. and another doctor came to my room to talk to me about putting me on Prednisone. But because I once had pancreasitis, which they suspected was caused by Prednisone, they wanted me to remain in the hospital for a day longer so they could observe the drug's reaction on me. I was scheduled to be discharged the next day after dialysis and I was very reluctant to remain in the hospital even for one more day. We then decided to wait till the next week, which would also give the radiation a chance to work.

The next day, after dialysis, I was discharged from the hospital. Although I was feeling somewhat better than when I came in, my knees were not doing too well and the rest of my joints were still quite painful.

On Thursday, April 3, 1980, my arthritis was much worse so that, when I was taken off dialysis, I was admitted back to T4E ward, where they gave me my first 20 mg. dose of Prednisone. A few hours later I began feeling better and had a good night's sleep.

On Friday I was feeling very much better and received my second 20 mg. dose of Prednisone. It upset my stomach, so I got Basajel, which cleared it up. I felt so well that I got up and walked with my crutches on my own. This was the first time in three weeks that I was able to get out of the wheelchair without help. I walked to the Day Room, watched TV for a while, than on the way back ran into the doctor—who was jubilant to see that my joints were so much better. When I got back to my room I was a bit exhausted because my muscles were still weak.

On Saturday, after dialysis, Stephanie wheeled me back to the ward where I got dressed and got a small bottle of Prednisone. Then we both walked out of the hospital on my discharge.

Going back and forth from my home to the hospital for my dialysis treatments three times a week was no longer a problem for me. My joints were about ninety percent pain free, my movements were more limber and my morale was sky high.

Five days later, the doctor reduced my Prednisone from 20 mg. to 15 mg. per day.

Two weeks later, my Prednisone was reduced to 12½ mg. per day, with no reduction in my pain-free motions.

In May, I made arrangements with the nurses in the unit to get dialyzed on Friday afternoon instead of Saturday so that Stehanie and I could attend my nephew Raymond's wedding in Massachusetts. We went in my nephew-in-law's car, with his wife Linda, my niece, and my sister Dorothy, the mother of the groom. It was a four-hour drive each way and the wedding reception lasted till 6 P.M. We got home in the evening. This was my first long-distance trip since my kidney failure and my stamina was surprisingly as normal as everyone else's.

Since I had been on Prednisone my arthritis had been under very good control, and I was now down to 7½ mg. per day. On July 2, 1980 the doctor again reduced it, this time to 10 mg. every other day. The reason for the 10 mg. every other day, instead of 5 mg. every day, was because it had been found over the years that, when Prednisone was taken every other day instead of every day, there was a great reduction in the side-effects, which were the "moonface" appearance and the bone decalcification. Because I was especially worried about my bones which held the hip prosthesis, this was delightful news to hear. Therefore I was eager to cooperate fully with this every-other-day regimen.

Unfortunately this new regimen had a roller-coaster effect

on my athritis. On the first day after taking 10 mg. of Prednisone, I felt very well, but on the second day there was a steep decline into pain and stiffness. The doctor suggested that I give my body more time to adjust to it. Even if I had to increase the dosage, in the long run, it would still be better to take the higher dosage every other day than to take a smaller dosage every day.

I increased my Prednisone to 15 mg. every other day and, though the roller-coaster effect still prevailed, the downward decline was gradually growing less steep, and the pain and stiffness that did come were kept at bay with Tylenol and Darvon.

Although my spine had become shrunken, bent and distorted, reducing my height from 5'9½" down to 5'6", and my artificial hip joints kept getting more unstable and my eyesight kept deteriorating with cataracts, I was still very convinced that the struggle for survival was well worth it. I now found that I understood myself and the world a lot better.

As an optimist about the future of the world, I believe the people of the world will soon become tired of being manipulated by the greedy, and they will become angry enough to replace the insanity that dominates us with a sane way of sharing the earth's bountiful resources, which includes trees and flowers. But at that time I had no premonition that even the sight of trees and flowers would be taken from me.

Chapter 10

While I was still able to get around, Stephanie and I would visit friends and relatives, but mostly we went in the evenings to my brother Richard's house. Richard and his wife Carole and their two children, Markie and Keith, and their dog Peppie lived in a home not far from where we lived, and we talked on all manner of subjects and watched TV. Then, after I had my stomach surgery, Stephanie and I did practically no traveling outside our own home, not even to go to the movies as we used to do. Since Stephanie did not want to go out alone, we got cable TV instead.

But the trouble was my eyesight was becoming so blurred with cataracts that I could no longer see the movies on our TV set, nor was I able to read or write anymore.

I went to the V.A. Eye Clinic to have them change the prescription on my still new eyeglasses. The doctor said my cataracts were getting worse and new eyeglasses would not help. In desperation I answered an ad and bought myself a pair of black plastic eye glasses with tiny pin holes to look through. They enabled me to read, even though it was at a slow pace, and I even watched TV with them and used them continuously for these purposes. It was the best twenty-three-dollar investment I had ever made.

Every couple of months I went to the Eye Clinic and every doctor that examined my eyes told me they were not yet ripe for surgery. I had talked to many patients who had cataract surgery and they told me that, except for the slight discomfort from the Lydicaine needles, the surgery was nothing, no pain or anything, and they were able eventually to read again. I told the opthalmologist that I needed my eyes for reading and writing and would like to get the surgery there and then. He said the hospital's philosophy was that it would be immoral to operate on a patient who was still able to see well enough to get around. When a patient's eyesight became very bad, then the risk of surgery was worth it. I asked him about the risks. He said that about five percent did not respond well, but ninety-five percent did. But these statistics also covered people who had other eye diseases besides cataracts.

"How are my eyes in that regard?" I asked.

"Your eyes are healthy, so the risks for you are lower."

"Well, that sounds like good news for me," I said. "In that case, couldn't I get my surgery earlier?"

"I'm afraid not," the doctor said. "It goes back to what I have already said, this is hospital policy."

If I had been able to afford it, I would have gone to an outside opthalmologist, but since I could not, I reconciled myself to waiting, and reading and writing at a crawling pace.

On one of my periodic Eye Clinic appointments, an opthalmologist was examining my eyes and stumbling over himself. He wore glasses and had a flabby body that looked like it was covered with jiggling baby fat. He moved slowly and clumsily, as if he were totally exhausted, though he was only in his thirties. When he went to his desk, he almost lost his balance over his swivel chair before he sat down to write something on my chart, and began breathing heavily from that little exertion. He had practically no coordination and was completely discombobulated. If there was ever a person out of shape, he was it. I looked at Stephanie, who was also in the room, and she looked at me as if to say, "Is he for real?" We were just too astonished to believe our eyes.

I asked him, "Are you a surgeon?"

He answered, "Yes I am."

Stephanie and I again exchanged incredulous glances.

When we left his office, we discussed this doctor on our way home, and among other things Stephanie said, "How come the hospital allows a doctor like that to operate on people?"

"I don't know," I said. "Apparently they have very low standards."

Finally, a couple of months later on a Thursday afternoon in July, 1981, I was admitted to the hospital for blood tests, EKG and chest X-ray in preparations for cataract surgery.

Monday morning was my eye surgery day so I got up early and washed up and was eager and ready to go to the O.R. at 8 A.M. But when 8 o'clock came I asked the nurse if they had forgotten about me. She said that they had sent a patient ahead of me and I would have to wait until he came out. I was greatly disappointed.

Dr. S. had been one of the optholmalogists who had examined my eyes on at least three occasions, including the last one at which the decision to operate was made. He was an intelligent, well-coordinated and competent doctor and I had a lot of confidence in him. He controlled all the preparations for the surgery, and the clumsy doctor was often by his side, but the clumsy doctor was just an appendage to Dr. S., so I paid no attention to him. I felt secure that I was in good hands with Dr. S.

Anyway, it was not till noon, when the dinner trays were being distributed, that the nurse came to my room with a stretcher and told me they were ready for me. I got on the stretcher and was wheeled to the hallway just outside the

Operating Room door. I was in a good mood because soon I would be able to see and read clearly again.

Dr. S. told me not to worry and that everything would be fine.

With a smile I said, "Hey, I'm not worried. I'm happy to be getting my eyes fixed."

I was wheeled into the O.R. and transferred from the stretcher onto the table. There was a very sophisticated movie camera set up over the table, and after I was covered with green sterile cloth so that only my left eye was exposed, the cameraman focused his equipment, then the surgery began. First my eye was washed with some solution, then someone from behind my head held a needle on a syringe and jabbed it into my cheek just under my eye and twisted it in various directions and I screamed at the terrible pain that felt like a knife stabbing me. Then the needle moved to another site and I screamed again. "No more, no more!" I kept screaming as the needle went to a third sight. Then my eye became numb and the rest of the needle injections were painless. After that the surgery began, and I felt some slight tugging sensations. Although there were at least a half dozen people around me including the cameraman and his assistant, only the low, monotonous buzzing sounds from the camera could be heard. Finally, the operating doctor behind me began to speak, "Whew, it's hot in here! Isn't it hot in here?" Nobody answered him. Tranquilized as I was, I had become suddenly horror-stricken to hear that it was the voice of the clumsy, uncoordinated doctor with the baby fat who was actually cutting into my eye. I had been instructed not to move my head during surgery and I did not want to have my eye destroyed by this fool of a doctor if I created a commotion while the surgery was in progress. I therefore did not move or speak and just hoped that through some miracle the eye would survive the surgery.

Dr. Clumsy continued complaining about the heat and Dr. S., who was on the left side of my head, said that the temperature in the room was comfortable. Then a moment later, Dr. S. said, "Why are you using that stitch?"

Dr. Clumsy said, "I learned that stitch from Dr. X."

"That stitch is no longer being used," Dr. S. said. "If you should develop a snag you'd be in deep trouble."

Then a few minutes later, Dr. Clumsy made a soft intonation that sounded like "Whoops." This was followed by what seemed like some commotion behind me, which I perceived was Dr. S. now physically helping Dr. Clumsy out of some problem, and nobody spoke. A few minutes later it felt calmer as the surgery resumed. I asked from under the covers, "What happened?" but nobody answered me.

I could hear Dr. S. intermittantly directing Dr. Clumsy in medical language that was mostly inaudible to me.

The operation continued for an inordinately long time, and I was beginning to feel some discomfort in my eye and my back was aching from lying in one position for so long. Yet, I stoically endured it all and did not move until the operation was completed two and a half hours after it had begun.

A bulging bandage was placed over my eye, the covers were removed from my face and with my right eye I dimly saw the movie camera and the green-clad people around me who transferred me from the table to the stretcher. Then I was moved to an adjoining Recovery Room where a cheerful nurse took my blood pressure and, since I was in a good mood because the surgery was finally over, I joked with her. A half hour later, I was moved to the ward and Stephanie was there in the hallway waiting for me with a happy smile on her face. The doctors had told her the operation went well.

I was transferred to my bed and was feeling a considerable amount of pain in my bandaged eye, but I felt better when

Stephanie and I held hands. Nevertheless, the pain not only continued, but its intensity increased to the point where I could no longer bear it. I asked Stephanie if there was a nurse nearby, and said that I needed a pain-killer. Stephanie went to the nurses' station to tell them, and a nurse told Stephanie that she would bring it to me. An hour later, the nurse finally gave me the pain-killer and it did not immediately work on me. Stephanie told me that my right eye, which was not operated on, was also swollen and black and blue.

When my supper tray arrived, I was too sick to eat anything. Stephanie managed to get a few spoonfuls into me and I dozed off in the middle of chewing and had to be roused each time it happened. The pain-killer I had taken was now working on me and I was too groggy and numb to feel the pain. All I wanted to do was sleep, sleep, sleep.

When I awoke about an hour later with much of the pain in the eye back, the supper tray was gone and Stephanie was still there sitting at my bedside. "How do you feel?" she asked.

Besides the pain, my whole body and my disposition were full of miseries, and I sarcastically said, "Lousy." All my answers to her were short and resentful. I just wanted to lie there in my profound misery and be left alone without any annoyance whatsoever from anyone, not even from Stephanie, whom I loved.

Stephanie felt hurt by this short-shrift treatment and it added more fuel to my miseries. I cursed the son-of-a-bitch in the Operating Room who caused me all this terrible pain. This was more than I had bargained for, and far more than any cataract patient I had talked to ever had to endure. I was unnecessarily brutalized and I was angry as hell.

The next day my eye was still very painful and I got more pain-killers and, except for going to the bathroom and eating very little from my three trays, I slept like the dead. When

Stephanie arrived in the evening, I was a little more alert but still full of miseries and with not a very civil disposition.

On Wednesday I went to dialysis on a stretcher. I weighed 108 pounds when I got on the machine, and 105 when I got off. I slept through most of the six-hour run. The pain in my eye was reducing itself down to a tolerable level, and I no longer asked for pain-killers. On the following day I felt much better and started walking around with my Canadian crutches. Then on Friday, I went home with Stephanie on a weekend pass. At home Stephanie gave me the three different eye drops, four times a day, that I was getting in the hospital.

Early Monday morning, Stephanie got me back to the hospital. The doctors that had been examining my eye everyday since the surgery now told me it was beginning to look good and that I could go home on a discharge. Stephanie left her place of employment at noon and came to the hospital to take me home.

She continued giving me the three eye drops four times a day and changing the bandage. She then told me that a piece of the white part of the eye, the sclera, had been torn away, giving an oval shape to my pupil. She drew a sketch of it on a piece of paper to show me how it looked, and said that she did not say anything about it in the beginning because she thought it was only a temporary problem that would correct itself with time. At that point, we never suspected the disaster that would later come to that eye.

In dialysis the heart skips I had for the past three years were getting worse and the EKG showed some change. After the doctors had investigated my medical records they decided that the Digoxin I had been taking all that time was only aggravating the heart skips, so they told me to stop the Digoxin altogether. From then on I felt a lot better and my heart skips were greatly reduced, occurring only occasionally and only for short durations.

One day, after getting off dialysis, my blood pressure was down to 90/65. While eating supper at home I broke out in a cold sweat and became very weak and light-headed. Stephanie helped me get into bed and hand-fed the rest of my supper to me. I started to feel better after that. I had a few more such episodes and learned that the dialysis treatment had drained out all my nourishment. So from then on I had a bowl of chicken soup each time I got home.

The high blood pressure I had had for a couple of years before I got on dialysis was caused by my failing kidneys. When the kidneys stopped functioning and I went on dialysis, my blood pressure went back down to my normal 120/70. But occasionally dialysis would remove too much fluid from my body causing my blood pressure to drop below normal, resulting in a whooziness when I would stand up. But it was quickly corrected after I had had the best medicine in the world, a bowl of hot chicken soup. I wonder how many lives could be saved if all the pharmaceutical firms were turned into chicken soup factories.

Two months after my cataract operation, I was fitted with a soft porous contact lens. When the optician placed the lens on my eye, I barely detected anything being in my eye whatsoever, and—lo and behold—my vision immediately returned to 20/20 and a whole new world was opened up to me. Everything appeared bright with colors and in sharpness of detail. I saw Stephanie clearly for the first time in over a year and that expanded my great delight into sheer ecstasy! It was incredible! All my life I had been living with 20/20 vision and I just took it for granted! Not until I had lost my eyesight and then got it back did I realize how vibrantly beautiful and delightful the world actually was.

I wanted to continue wearing the lens but the optician said it was only a test lens and he would have to order one like it, and also have it tinted over the area that would cover the missing sclera in my eye to prevent too much light from getting in. Consequently, Stephanie and I left the Eye Clinic a bit disappointed but optimistic about the future.

In the interim, the ophthalmologist had scheduled me for cataract surgery on my right eye. I was admitted on a Thursday and had the pre-op tests done. Then, after dialysis, I went home on a weekend pass and returned Sunday evening.

Monday morning I went to the O.R. Dr. A., an ophthalmologist who I had gotten to know and in whom I had confidence, did the surgery. Those dreadful needles that I had had in my first cataract surgery were inserted so skillfully and gently that I barely felt any pain. When my eye was completely "blocked," the surgery began and twenty-three minutes later it was completed, and when I got back to the ward Stephanie saw that I was all smiles and I felt like a million dollars. Stephanie was amazed by the sharp contrast between this cataract surgery and the other one performed by Dr. Clumsy. When my supper tray arrived I had a good appetite and ate everything on my tray to Stephanie's and my happy satisfaction.

Two days later, as I was being dialyzed, I noticed a shadow in the lower part of my left eye, the eye which had been done by Dr. Clumsy. At first I thought the shadow may have been caused by some mucous. But after carefully wiping the eye with tissue I realized that it was still there. When I looked down the shadow was not visible, but when I looked up the shadow appeared like a half-risen black sun and, like Lady Macbeth, I shouted inside myself so no one else could hear me, "Out, damned spot! Out, I say!" over and over again to try to exorcise it out of my eye. Although I did not know what it was, I suspected that it was something ominous and I imagined all kinds of horrors. I brought it to the attention of my primary nurse and asked her to call the Eye Clinic.

When I got off dialysis Dr. A. examined the eye, then said, "You have a very serious problem."

I almost sank through the chair, and said, "Oh, Christ!"

Then he told me I had a detached retina. I asked him what that meant. He explained that the retina was peeling away in the back of my eye, like wallpaper, and elaborated on the function of the retina and suggested I submit to surgery to reattach it. Otherwise it would peel off altogether and become impossible to reattach and would leave me sightless in that eye. I was stunned by the impact of possibly losing an eye, and my mind sputtered down to a dull low speed for a moment, but soon it resumed its normal revolutions per minute and I realized that surgery was my only hope.

Dr. A. called in a team of three retina specialists, including one woman. They examined my left eye and said that this operation was more complex than a simple cataract operation. Therefore it would have to be done under general anasthesia.

In late afternoon I talked to the anesthesiologist and made it clear to him that I could not move my head back to accept the breathing tube through my throat. He said they would try a soft tube through my nose and have a doctor standing by to perform a tracheotomy just in case.

At 8 A.M. the following morning I was in the Operating Room. For half an hour they tried to insert one tube after another into my nose and windpipe, spraying my nose with a bitter numbing solution, and each time they tried I choked from lack of air and was unable to speak to let them know that I could not breathe. I found that my hands had been tied at my sides so that I was totally helpless and unable to protect myself from my unwiting assassins—who would later apologize to Stephanie, "We're sorry, but he unexpectedly died of heart failure."

Fortunately, through some miracle, the breathing tube slipped into my windpipe and I began to breathe life-saving air, and then the anesthesia rendered me senseless. When I woke up five and a half hours later and I spent one and one half hours in the Recovery Room, I was told the surgery went well and I smiled. When I got back to my bed, Stephanie was also smiling happily.

But as the days passed, our happiness changed to suspense-filled anguish. Dr. Alice C., one of the three retina surgeons, who had been examining my eyes every day since the surgery, had found a small amount of fluid under the reattached retina and kept observing it daily, hoping it would eventually dissipate of its own accord. If it did not, there was the possibility that the fluid would again detach the retina, therefore I would again need surgery on that eye.

When it looked like the fluid had been reduced a bit, I was discharged from the hospital with a cloud still hanging over my head, and I was told to come for weekly clinic visits.

Since Dr. C. worked mostly at the major local hospital, that was where most of my clinic appointments were. The waiting room was always crowded and each clinic visit lasted from four to six hours. The fluid under the retina fluctuated in terms of the size of the puddle, but basically the trend was toward a bigger build-up. Dr. C. called into the room a top retina specialist, Dr. Q., who was also her superior. Dr. Q. examined my eye with his lighted eyepiece for a few seconds, then said, "Perfect," and started to leave the room. I immediately said, "Dr. C. thought she saw some fluid." Taken aback Dr. Q. again looked into my eye and searched around but was unable to find the fluid. Dr. C. told him, exactly where to look. He finally found the spot and told Dr. C. to search for a tiny hole and he left the room. She looked very carefully but could not find any. Finally it was decided that a laser beam be used to isolate the puddle. We went into another room where I was seated on one side of the laser machine and Dr. C. on the other side of it. I asked her if it would be painful, and she said she would adjust the strength of the beam so there would be only slight discomfort. As she was getting ready to adjust it, Dr. Q. barged into the room, told Dr. C. to move and sat down in her place. He told me not to move my eyes, then he fired a beam, and I felt a sharp pain and I wanted to shift my eyes away from the beam. But my strong desire to save my eye outweighed the pain and I stoicaly kept my eyes perfectly still and endured the steady bombardment of laser beams that Dr. Q. kept firing at me as if he were in a penny arcade. It was only a short period but it felt as if it would never end. I was greatly consoled when it was finally over, although some residual pain still hung on.

On the way home Stephanie told me that when I had told Dr. Q. that Dr. C. thought she saw some fluid under my retina, Stephanie saw Dr. C. put her hand over her mouth as if I had let the cat out of the bag and her subservience to the Big Retina Diety was being put in jeopardy. It was ironic to me that an intelligent and compassionate person like Dr. C., who was highly skilled and had empathy with her patients, should allow herself to be subservient to what I felt was a cold, calculating walking encyclopedia. Then Stephanie asked me about the laser beam, and I told her that Dr. Q. had burned tiny spots around the fluid puddle to form scar tissue that would keep the fluid from spreading in the hope that the puddle would eventually dry up.

A week later, we were back at the Eye Clinic. Dr. C. saw that more fluid had accumulated under the retina and Dr. Q. said there had to be a tiny hole somewhere that was letting the fluid seep through. After a considerable search, the minute hole was found. I was told that I needed surgery to close it up, otherwise the fluid buildup would eventually detach the retina again. Dr. C. said the surgery was not urgent, but I should think about it for at least a week. My emotions were in turmoil. The horrors of my first retina operation still gnawed on me like a sharp tooth painfully embedded into my very soul, along with the anger at Dr. Clumsy, who was the source of my present pain and anguish, and the knowledge that I would lose my left eye if I did not submit to the wrath of another operation. It all weighed heavily on me.

At home Stephanie and I pondered my dilemma over and over again, and each time we concluded that, despite all the horror I would have to face, my eye was too precious to lose. Therefore our decision was that I would wait at least a week before I would give my consent to have the retina surgery.

But three days later while I was in dialysis, Dr. S. came to the unit and told me my surgery was scheduled for the following day. I was appalled by this sudden decision, even before I had given my consent, since I had planned to wait at least a week. Dr. S. said that Dr. Q. had a free day the following day and was available to do the retina surgery, and that it was urgent for me to get it done as soon as possible. I knew he was lying about the urgency of the operation and that the real reason I was being rushed through was for the sole convenience of Dr. Q. Since Dr. Q. was reportedly one of the top specialists in the field of retina surgery, Dr. S. said I should not miss this fine opportunity to get the best. I assumed that Dr. Q.'s excellent reputation was well deserved and I agreed to accept the surgery the next day, although I resented the way it had been suddenly foisted upon me.

On the following morning, I was up at 6 and washed up, then had an EKG and was ready before 9 o'clock. At 9 A.M. I was in the Operating Room. Dr. Q., Dr. C., Dr. S., a nurse, a cameraman and a woman anesthesiologist were present. The anesthesiologist put an I.V. into my right arm and took my blood pressure. We had already agreed that I would get a local rather than a general anesthesia. Dr. Q. asked me to look up and he injected Lydicaine under my eye ball and I let out a cry at the terrible pain. As he continued injecting around my eye he was also lecturing to the doctors about what to avoid touching with the needle punctures. When my eye was completely numb Dr. Q. began the surgery and continued giving information to the other doctors. The operation went smoothly. There was no question about Dr. Q.'s abilities, he was a very good surgeon and his reputation as a top retina specialist was indeed well deserved. When the operation was finished Dr. Q. left amid a round of applause and compliments. Dr. S. put antibacterial salve over my eye and bandaged it. Then I went to the Recovery Room for a while, and finally to my room.

In bed I had to lay on my back with my head raised at least thirty degrees to keep the fluid pressure in the eyes down. This I also had to do after my first retina operation and I had developed bedsores on my lower spine that were still not healed. This time I had to begin with painful bedsores and continued aggravating them through the second retina healing. Lying on my back I was not allowed to turn on my sides, but Dr. S. told me I could get up for bathroom privileges. But in the evening when I put on my call light because I had a bowel movement coming on, the orderly came over and told me I was not allowed to get up. I told him that I wanted to see a nurse. A few minutes later a nurse came and told me the same thing. I asked her if she had read my chart and she said she did not but the first shift nurses had briefed all the second shift nurses that I was not to get up out of bed. I later talked to another nurse and two female orderlies who told me the same thing. Because of my rigid spine I could not roll over on my side while my upper torso was raised at thirty degrees. I decided against having to go through the agonizing process of trying to get the bed pan under me. Therefore, I held my bowels until the urge was gone, but I still felt some discomfort in my lower stomach.

When the midnight shift came in I explained my situation to the head nurse, who was a kindly middle-aged woman, and I told her how I had pleaded with the nurses to read my chart and asked her to please read it. She said she would be glad to read it. A few minutes later she returned to my room and read the doctor's instructions. Among the list of other orders was written that I was allowed bathroom privileges. She apologized for what had happened to me and said she could not understand why so many nurses did not bother to read the doctor's actual orders. She fully agreed with my complaints. She asked me if I would like to get up now and I told her that I did not feel the urge to go, but that I would get up to try. She cranked down the head of the bed then helped me up to a sitting position on the side of the bed. With my crutches I went to the bathroom, but it turned out to be a dry run. When I returned to my bed my worries about my bathroom privileges were now gone and I slept soundly until 6 A.M., at which time I felt the urge to go. This time, when I called for help, an orderly helped me out of bed without question and things ran smoothly again. I washed up, then at 7 A.M. I was taken by wheel chair to Building #2 for my dialysis. I had to lie on my back for six hours on the painful bedsores that were draining small drops of pus and that had to be covered with gauze, which increased my pain. The nurses tried to assuage the pain by placing an air-filled doughnut under my back, but it did not work. Then they taped a wide piece of sponge over the area and the pain was greatly alleviated.

Four days later I was discharged from the hospital.

Then two days after that, while in dialysis, my eye, the eye that had already experienced three operations, began aching severely. It felt as though someone was crushing the entire eye ball and the pain was growing intolerable. The nurse phoned the Eye Clinic and an ophthalmologist, within minutes, came up to the unit and carefully examined my eye with his bright light. He said he did not see anything wrong. I asked him if I had an infection and he answered in the negative, then he added, "The buckle was a little too tight around the retina, but it should loosen up with time."

I wiped mucous out of my eye, and said, "But there is a lot of mucous coming out of my eye."

The ophthalmologist did not think it was anything to worry about and attributed it to irritation.

A couple of days later I went to the Eye Clinic and another ophthalmologist told me that the pain was caused when the recently cut nerves had grown back together again and protested the tight buckle, but the pain should gradually go away. In the meantime, my right eye, from which the cataract was removed in twenty-three minutes by Dr. A., had no complications and the eyesight in it would eventually be 20/20 with corrective glasses.

The pain in my left eye continued for hours at a time and would spread into a big headache and down to the back of my neck. Later the eye began to ooze more mucous, and gradually the pain grew less intense.

I had an appointment with Dr. C. at the local major hospital clinic, and after three hours of waiting I got into her office. She examined my eye and said that I again had fluid under my retina and another small hole. I also had an infection, for which I was given medication for the first time since over a week of mucous discharge, which the V.A. doctors had known about. She also added that if the infection was in the buckle, then the buckle would have to be removed. I was distressed and angry and left her office feeling like a zombie. As Stephanie drove me home she cursed the doctors for putting me through all that pain and still not saving the eye. We both vented our anger and after a while felt a little better.

Two days later while in dialysis, a culture was taken of the mucous, which now was turning yellow. I was already getting antibiotics and now they were going to identify the bacteria to determine what kind of antibiotics I was supposed to get!

The night after that, I woke up with a black shadow over one third of the eye. Then a day later the retina was completely detached and I was totally blind in one eye. Yet, instead of being outraged, I felt a strange sense of relief. For me pain was the name of the game and I was too tired and broken-down to play anymore. After my last visit to the major hospital clinic the handwriting was already on the wall predicting the inevitable. I went through a great deal of hell trying to save the eye and now it was finally all over. The eye was gone and nothing more could be done for it and I was glad that the goddamn nightmare was finally ended.

On my next Eye Clinic visit at the V.A. the ophthalmologist told me what I already knew, that my retina was completely detached. Also he said that the chances of getting it reattached successfully were almost nil. I told him that I would not submit to any more eye surgery anyway. He prescribed new eye drops and oral antibiotics for the infection.

Stephanie and I went to a law firm and instituted a malpractice suit against Dr. Clumsy, who was still practicing at the hospital as well as at his own private office. I do not hate him, it is not his fault that his abilities render him incompetent, it is just that he should not be allowed to operate on patients any more than drunks should be allowed to drive, and if they do harm to anyone, they should pay for it.

Gradually my arthritis flared up and, despite increasing my Prednisone dosage under doctor's supervision, my joints were terribly swollen and I found it almost impossible to function.

My disposition was atrocious and I was surly to everyone, including Stephanie. At the hospital I was hostile and sarcastic and complained to everyone I came in contact with about how I had lost my eye and cursed the damn quacks and the hospital. I also complained about all the little annoyances in the dialysis unit that had before and even then plagued me. I was just simply and unequivocally angry, and I ranted and raved at everyone, and in between, I seethed and brooded like a pent-up bull.

Prior to my eye loss, I had been meeting with a V.A. psychologist for one and one half hours every week. He was a soft-spoken young man with a short beard who had the facility to understand his patients. We went through a battery of question-and-answer tests. My vision was too poor for me to read the tests and the psychologist, Dr. K., read out each question and I answered them orally. After some weeks, the tests were all completed for the computer to analyze. Dr. K. told me I was well adjusted and adequately capable of coping with my problems, despite all my incredible trials and tribulations.

He said he found me to be an unusual person and asked me if I would not mind continuing our weekly sessions. I was enthusiastic about continuing because I learned a lot and considered Dr. K. to be brilliant in his field. He and I had a good rapport.

He had a tape recorder and wanted to know more about my background. I told him how we had lived through the 1930's Depression in Bridgeport, and the fights my father and mother had over lack of money, his long layoff from his job and his humiliation at having his family living on welfare. My mother, my brother Joe and I would pick up the weekly food box because my father was too ashamed to do so. My father, who was a healthy man wanting desperately to support his family, was reduced to idleness. He would often take Joe and me to the city dumps to salvage things we could use and collected aluminum pots, copper wire, brass and zink and rags that we sold to the junk yard. Also we would pick up wood-tar blocks for firewood where streets were being torn up to remove trolley tracks. At the same time the wealthy were feeding sirloin steaks to their poodles, which I saw in a magazine I found at the city dumps.

In those days my brother Joe and I were inseparable companions. We went fishing, swimming and playing with the gang of kids in the neighborhood, exploring the wide range of forests on the outskirts north of the city and sometimes getting into fights with other gangs. But there never was any real violence and there were no knives or guns involved.

But the saddest note to me, which I still regretted bitterly and which there was no way to undo, was that Joe and I had treated our younger brother Bill abominably. Billy, as we had called him, was a happy kid with a kind and sensitive disposition and everyone liked him. But because he was somewhat younger than Joe and I, he did not fit in with our wide-ranging activities. Each time Joe and I would leave the house Billy would be there trailing behind us. To get rid of him we would tell him to go home and then throw stones at him when he refused. But because we did not want to harm him, we threw stones low, not wanting to even hit his legs. He drew back, then crying bitter tears turned to go home, and Joe and I were free to go on our way. How cruel and insensitive we were when we were young.

It never occurred to us that he was lonely and that by so callously rejecting him we had hurt him severely many times over.

When I grew up, I discovered that my father was a very interesting person. He and I had long discussions about almost everything under and beyond the sun. He told me that he felt badly about his inability to communicate with his children during their growing up years because he had not fully mastered the English language. His first language was Slovak, and when he tried to convey his thoughts to someone, the exact meaning would become lost in translation. The result was that people would sometimes get the wrong meaning and would think he was being rude and insulting.

Anyway, over the years, my father had become somewhat

more articulate and he and I continued our discussions. Mostly we would drink beer and sit in beach chairs in my back yard. We covered astronomy, philosophy, paleontology, sociology, politics, history and current affairs. I was surprised by his wide range of knowledge and understanding and his above-average intelligence, something that had not been very discernible from his broken English. I found the discussions very stimulating and I learned a lot from him.

When my father became bedridden in his last weeks of life, Stephanie and I brought him to our home to take some of the burden from my mother, who was taking care of him. Though his mind was lucid, he spoke very little and, when he did speak, it was mostly in monosyllables. But at night, he would wake up screaming and saying in Slovak that he was being bitten by swarms of insects. When I put on the light in his room his hands were frantically brushing away the imaginary insects. After I assured him that there were no insects, he calmed down and slowly scratched his itching chest while I scratched his back till he felt better. It was at periods like that, when my father would become delirious, that he did some talking, mostly in his Slovak language which I understood clearly.

One day while I was shaving him, he spoke in English and said, "The time comes quick?" He was telling me how short life was. When one considers that it takes a lifetime to become wise, life is indeed short.

During my sessions with the psychologist, Dr. K., I had been releasing all my guilts and regrets and told how they still disturbed me whenever these incidents entered my mind. Dr. K. told me that I should measure my shortcomings against my assets. He asked me for one asset. For the life of me I could not think of any. Then Dr. K., who had gotten to know me, said, "Here's a few: I like people, I haven't found a person that I hated, I always see the good in people. I like myself for my political activism." Then he asked me to think of more. "I feel good about my writing," I said. "I value my fighting spirit. I have a good relationship with my wife, I love her. Glad I bought an electrically operated bed. I feel good about my work as a shop steward. I feel good about the lawsuit I won and the precedent it set. I'm kind. I'm glad I joined the Library for the Blind to help me read books on cassette tapes. I'm glad I bought plastic eyeglasses with pinholes. I feel good that my wife and I went to Cuba in 1960 to observe the people's revolution firsthand. I feel good that I write letters to newspapers to express my opinions. I am a survivor. I am at peace with myself...."

Dr. K. had opened up many new insights about myself that were very helpful and enlightening to me. Our sessions ended and I saw him on occasions when he would come up to dialysis to see how I was doing.

But after I had lost my eye and vented my anger at everyone, he came up to see me and we talked about my anger and we went back to our weekly sessions. I told him that my arthritis was very painful, making it almost impossible to function as a self-sufficient person, and that the arthritis flare-ups were usually associated with frustrating crisis. He thought that by releasing my anger I reduced the built-up tensions in myself, and suggested that I become more assertive toward staff people who give me a runaround. After a few sessions Dr. K. had taught me how to overcome my pain by meditation, and my anger was gone and the sessions ended.

I was back to being my old self again and gradually the huge flare-up of my arthritis had gone down to tolerable levels that allowed me to function more comfortably.

Everything was going fine for me. Then one morning as I was walking toward the dialysis unit my crutches slipped on a wet spot and I went crashing to the floor. I was helped up to my feet and was surprised that I was not seriously hurt.

Then several months later I fell again. This time I had

pain in my hips that lasted a while. Because I had still not received my glasses, I was unable to see water on the floor, and I walked with great caution and fear until I finally got them. From then on, with good vision in my right eye, I had the ability to avoid water spills in my path.

In January 1982, Stephanie got laid off from her job and joined the other millions of unemployed workers who were victims of Reaganomics.

One thing that surprised me above all else in this hospital was finding many nurses, whom I thought were above such things, expressing the view that, because medical treatment for veterans was "free," veterans should not complain about their treatment. This attitude was held by even some of the more dedicated nurses who did their job well. Thus, patients caught in bureaucratic bunglings had to continue suffering the consequences of these bunglings because practically nobody was willing to stick his or her neck out to make corrections—expecially since they felt that the patients were freeloaders.

Such distorted values, of course, are caused by our competitive, dog-eat-dog society where the climate is conducive to the growth of conflicts, resentments and hatreds that subconsciously effects us all.

Therefore I feel the need to emphasize the fact that veterans are not freeloaders. Federal laws entitle veterans who had served during wartime to free medical treatment. But nowhere in these laws does it stipulate that these patients must also accept abuses. Veterans have every right to complain when these abuses occur, and they definitely do occur.

Furthermore, I believe that every person in this country should be entitled to the same socialized medicine that the veterans receive.

Unfortunately, under our current competitive system, socialized medicine would be subjected to many abuses and corruptions and would leave a lot to be desired. Still, it would be better than our present, chaotic, out-of-control system.

However, in this highly technological period in our society wherein every aspect of our economy will ultimately become computerized and robotized, private ownership of industries will become impractical and they will therefore also have to be socialized to make them work. Only then, when the entire country is socialized, will socialized medicine find itself in a friendly climate where it will operate efficiently and humanely.

In the meantime my friend Jack Fernandez has had his own great burdens to bear. Shortly after one of his daughters had died, his wife succumbed to a stroke. But a year later he had remarried and settled down in his new wife's hometown in North Carolina, from which he still phones me once a week. I was delighted that he had the strength and the courage to put his life back together again.

I too was grateful for surviving all my life-threatening problems. The highly skilled doctors and kind nurses who constitute the majority of the hospital staff had helped me enormously. But it was my wife Stephanie, my very wonderful Florence Nightingale, who gave me the strength to fight all the impossible odds, that really made the difference. Love, it seems, can accomplish miracles. It stimulates the will to live and conquers disease through the mysterious mesmerization of mind over matter.

What is this endless stream of life all about? Life is in constant motion, dancing to the ghostly background noises of the universe, moving inexorably toward something that is still incomprehensible to us all, but which I believe is ultimately toward some worthy end.